Management of Spinal Cord Injury by Physiotherapist

(Site to Settlement)

Management of Spinal Cord Injury by Physiotherapist

(Site to Settlement)

Dilip Ambalal Patel
PhD PT (Rehab)
Formerly, Principal
Government Physiotherapy College
Government Spine Institute
Ahmedabad, Gujarat, India

Co-authors
Anjali Ravindra Bhise
PhD MPT (Cardiopulmonary)
Senior Lecturer and Principal In-Charge
Civil Hospital
Ahmedabad, Gujarat, India

Yagna Unmesh Shukla
PhD MPT (Musculoskeletal)
Senior Lecturer
Government Physiotherapy College
Government Spine Institute, Civil Hospital
Ahmedabad, Gujarat, India

Guest Editor
Dinesh Sorani
PhD BPT MPT

Foreword
MM Prabhakar

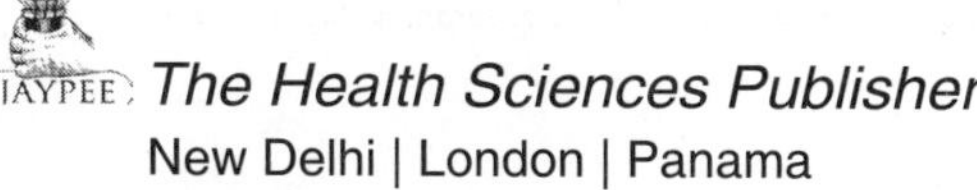

The Health Sciences Publisher
New Delhi | London | Panama

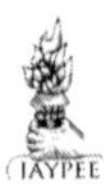

Jaypee Brothers Medical Publishers (P) Ltd

Headquarters

Jaypee Brothers Medical Publishers (P) Ltd
4838/24, Ansari Road, Daryaganj
New Delhi 110 002, India
Phone: +91-11-43574357
Fax: +91-11-43574314
Email: jaypee@jaypeebrothers.com

Overseas Offices

J.P. Medical Ltd
83 Victoria Street, London
SW1H 0HW (UK)
Phone: +44 20 3170 8910
Fax: +44 (0)20 3008 6180
Email: info@jpmedpub.com

Jaypee-Highlights Medical Publishers Inc
City of Knowledge, Bld. 235, 2nd Floor, Clayton
Panama City, Panama
Phone: +1 507-301-0496
Fax: +1 507-301-0499
Email: cservice@jphmedical.com

Jaypee Brothers Medical Publishers (P) Ltd
17/1-B Babar Road, Block-B, Shaymali
Mohammadpur, Dhaka-1207
Bangladesh
Mobile: +08801912003485
Email: jaypeedhaka@gmail.com

Jaypee Brothers Medical Publishers (P) Ltd
Bhotahity, Kathmandu
Nepal
Phone: +977-9741283608
Email: kathmandu@jaypeebrothers.com

Website: www.jaypeebrothers.com
Website: www.jaypeedigital.com

Inquiries for bulk sales may be solicited at: jaypee@jaypeebrothers.com

Management of Spinal Cord Injury by Physiotherapist (Site to Settlement)

First Edition: **2018**

ISBN 978-93-5270-269-5

Printed at Sanat Printers

Dedicated to

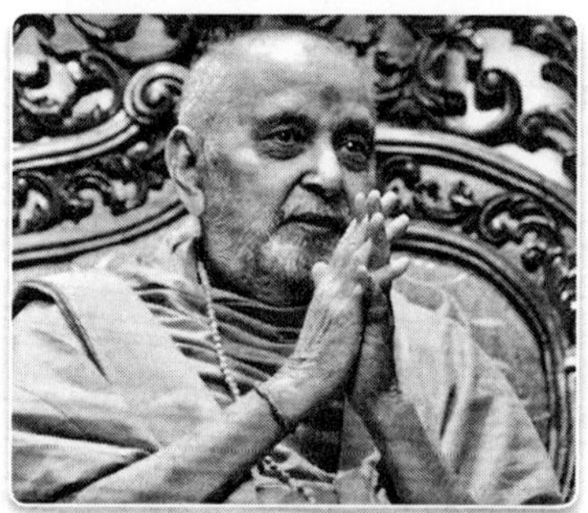

My Guru and God
His holiness late Pujya Pramukh Swami Maharaj

Foreword

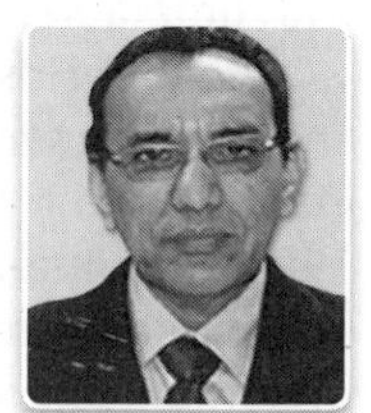

It is my pride and privilege to write this foreword as a Director of Government Spine Institute, Civil Hospital, Ahmedabad; Medical Superintendent, New Civil Hospital, Ahmedabad and Professor and Head, Department of Orthopedics, BJ Medical College, Civil Hospital, Ahmedabad, Gujarat.

I know all the authors very well. Professor Dr Dilip Patel has worked under me since 1992. He joined Civil Hospital as a clinical therapist in 1974. He was promoted to senior clinical therapist, senior lecturer and retired as a Principal, Government Physiotherapy College in 2007 and then joined Ahmedabad Institute of Medical Science, Ahmedabad. He has availed his PhD on Paraplegia Rehabilitation under my guidance. He has presented many scientific papers in the national conferences and has received awards as well. Dr Patel has travelled a lot and has visited many rehabilitation set-ups in India and abroad. Dr Patel is a sincere, sober, diligent and dedicated worker.

Mrs Anjali Ravindra Bhise—Senior Lecturer and Principal Government Physiotherapy College, Civil Hospital, Ahmedabad and Mrs Yagna Unmesh Shukla—Senior Lecturer and Administrative In-Charge of Rehabilitation Medicine Department - B1, Civil Hospital are also punctual, proactive, serious and solemn workers. They both did their Bachelor and Master in Physiotherapy. They joined as clinical therapist and were promoted as Lecturers and Senior Lecturers. They both have presented many scientific papers in the state and national conferences as well in a UK conference recently.

All the authors have vast experience of more than 25 years in the field of physiotherapy and rehabilitation. With their active involvement as rehabilitation team members for over 10,000 spinal cord injury patients at the Government Spine Institute, all are right professionals to write on this subject.

The authors have come up with an innovative idea. In the present era of Internet, where lots of information are available on net, this presentation with academics and actual activities, with pictures will help to perceive the problems and proceedings of treatment, not only to the professionals but also to the patients and people. The free flow of the book will hold the reader throughout and will also tempt to read and to revise repeatedly. There is a new novel concept of "Day cycle." The patients are prepared to plan and play the day-to-day activities with timetable.

The Civil Hospital is in 110 acres land, has many medical education and medical services programs. The Government Spine Institute was inaugurated by the then Prime Minister Shri Morarjibhai Desai in 1978. The ultra-modern building is disabled friendly (with ramp and lift), without architectural barriers. It is an 80-bedded hospital with Undergraduate and Postgraduate Physiotherapy and Prosthetic Orthotic Undergraduate colleges. It has better and bigger rehabilitation set-up with high tech machines, best structures and systems of functioning. Patients get holistic, highest order of rehabilitation services. Many fruitful academic and social supportive activities go on throughout the year. Many non-governmental organizations (NGOs) are involved to support the patients in their rehabilitation programs—emotionally, socially and financially and to provide them home-type atmosphere during their 4–6 months of stay. "We do not learn best, by memorizing facts about the subject, because reality is communal, we learn best by interacting with it." Many professionals come to learn and many to teach in the Government Spine Institute. It has become in a true sense an interactive learning center with an ideal service provider and an academic set-up.

Paraplegia and spinal injury patients were neglected in the past. "An ailment not to be treated" and they are "destined to die" was the writings in medical literature, until Dr Donald Munro of Boston, USA and Dr Ludwig Guttmann at Stoke Mandeville, UK, who did pioneering work for spinal cord injury (SCI) rehabilitation after the Second World War. The message spread all over the world and now many specialized such centers are serving SCI patients.

Body's structures, systems and its functioning with preventive medicine, curative-palliative medicine, and rehabilitation medicine with dimensions of IBR, OBR, CBR and CAHD are very well described in this book.

Authors have given special thought on the problems of patient's partner and caregiver. SCI needs long-term care and require lots of physical work of lifting and transferring. Also, they need constant emotional support. Caregivers get tired with the physical task and get emotionally exhausted. The book has included the topic of "caring the caregivers" with the biomechanical, psychosexual issues. Student's support services with "learners are good servers" if guided well, are also a good thought to present.

Mentioning about basic services of Orthopedics, Nursing, PT, OT, ST, P&O, MSW, Psychology, Vocational, NGO-related to SCI in the book is useful to many rehabilitation professionals.

Role of a self is important in the rehabilitation process of disabled in general and spinal cord injury patients in particular. Patients are "active achievers" of the "goal" rather than the "passive recipient" of rehabilitation services. At the Government Spine Institute, this principle is well observed and all patients are involved and integrated in their rehabilitation program.

Authors have divided the Section 3 into two major stages of SCI care—(1) Survival stage and (2) Settlement stage, which is a new concept of presentation.

This book will become "unique" with different sections. The style with the stuff of presentation will help to take the rehabilitation message of spinal cord injury for prevention and program of proceedings to the professionals (Medical, Nursing and Rehabilitation), also to the patients and people. The book is sure to serve the purpose.

MM Prabhakar
MS (Ortho)
Additional Director
Medical Education and Research
Gujarat State
Medical Superintendent
New Civil Hospital, Ahmedabad
Director
Government Physiotherapy College and Government Spine Institute
Civil Hospital, Ahmedabad
Professor and Head, Department of Orthopedics
BJ Medical College
Ahmedabad, Gujarat, India
President
Gujarat Nursing Council
Email: drmmprabhakar@gmail.com, paraplegiahospital@vsnl.net

Foreword

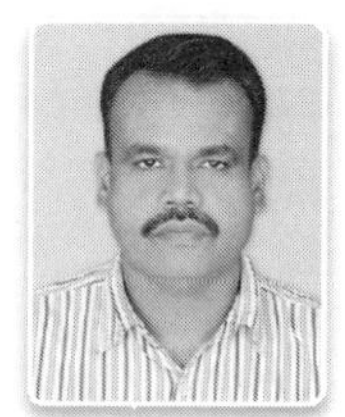

This book is written by Professor Dr Dilip Ambalal Patel and co-authors Mrs Anjali Ravindra Bhise and Mrs Yagna Unmesh Shukla.

I know all of them personally, as very good human beings and professionally, as dedicated clinicians, teachers, and administrators who have contributed a lot to physiotherapy profession.

I have been highly inspired by their work and there is a great impact of their professional knowledge and skills that they have shared with me.

I think with the help of this book, they will share knowledge, skills and a vast/varied experience of working with spinal cord injury and clinical reasoning with critical thinking skills with physiotherapy-rehabilitation students, teachers and clinical professionals across different parts of India and the globe.

I hope that this book will emerge as one of the most popular and best seller books in India and abroad.

Subhash M Khatri
MPT (Ortho) PhD (sports) FIAP
Principal
Dr APJ Abdul Kalam College of Physiotherapy
Pravara Institute of Medical Sciences
Ahmednagar, Maharashtra, India
Email: physiokhatri@gmail.com

Preface

Final year B Physio/M Physio students and the rehabilitation professionals are in need of learning and understanding of a good rehabilitation and resettlement process. At the Government Spine Institute, a good work of total/holistic restoration, resettlement program is being carried out for the Spinal Cord Injury patients; covering physical, mental, social, and vocational aspects. We combined "need and supply" principle and wrote this book.

This book contains initial medical and surgical interventions and then the resettlement process from "site of injury to settlement at home and work place". The students and the rehabilitation professionals will like "academics and actual actions".

The journey of writing this book is vivid. We all learned a lot—conceptualizing, gathering information, understanding book writing skills, indexing, correcting medical mistakes and English errors, where and how to place photographs, finding out publishers, finding strategy for marketing the book and finally finding out time to do the task from busy schedule. Book writing has improved our professional perceptions and image with importance.

During text writing, there were numerous problems and we solved them sitting together, talking on telephones and through emails (Thanks to the technology era).

We thank Professor Dr MM Prabhakar Sir, for his overall support, rehabilitation team at Government Spinal Institute, patients, students, M/s Jaypee Brothers Medical Publishers, and our family for supporting us constantly.

Book writing is a task like a marathon run—conceptualizing, deciding, determining, diligence, dedication, and directing—it took more than 3 years to reach the goal.

We suggest students and professionals to read the whole book at a stretch and refer the specialized area as and when needed. Please use the knowledge and perceptions for better care of SCI patients and imparting knowledge to the students.

Dilip Ambalal Patel
Anjali Ravindra Bhise
Yagna Unmesh Shukla

Acknowledgments

A book is a landmark and a light house for many students and staff to come into limelight. Writing a book needs enthusiasm, energy, efforts, and helping hands. This book will enhance the education and the present care of spinal cord injury (SCI) patients who were neglected in the past. This book is patient focused and we have described the scenario from "site to settlement" of SCI patients. Physiotherapy rehabilitation topics, including different disciplines, are covered in this book along with the rehabilitation process of SCI patients.

First and foremost, our gratitude to "God" for the spiritual support for preparing and presenting this book. Parents and professors, our second God. Parents who gave a birth as a Person and Professors gave birth as a Professional—words are not enough for their task of nourishing and nurturing. Our today's identity, image, importance, and income is because of them; we are indebted to them. Thanks to our family and friends for the favors. We have developed a "skill-to-steal" time from our family and reaching to iPad/computers for texting the text, thanks to them for bearing with us in this gesture of giving back to our profession.

Specifically speaking, Professor Dr MM Prabhakar Sir, a visionary and our mentor who believes in "Work is to be Worshiped"; inspired, insisted, allowed, and assisted with a care and concern for writing this book to help the students, staff, patients and people about the spinal cord injury for the management with actual activities. When he visited our home in Maryland, USA, he reminded me about the book writing project, which was planned in India 3 years before. We are thankful to him.

Credits to the caring and contributing co-authors: Mrs Anjali Ravindra Bhise and Mrs Yagna Unmesh Shukla. We have had nearly 25 years of association of working together, caring patients and teaching students. As rehabilitation team members, we have treated more than 10,000 SCI patients. This book is an outcome of our experience, which will be useful to the future caretaker professionals. We have good chemistry, comfortability, compatibility, and complementary values. We worked well for a satisfying, successful National Physiotherapy Conference, 2006. Right from the beginning, we had our dream and a desire to give a good book to the Physio-Rehab professionals, pupil, and patients on SCI rehabilitation program. We are happy to see our dream, a reality.

A special mention about our beloved students for contributing "two poems" related to the rehabilitation process of SCI patients. As such, this is a science book but subjective forces of Faith, Prayer, Love, Affection, and Kind words are utmost needed in the rehabilitation process. It will harness patient's energy, enthusiasm, and efforts. Dinesh Sorani is, at present, serving as a Senior Lecturer at Government Physiotherapy College, Jamnagar, Gujarat. His "Climb up the Rope of Hope" poem is effective to put efforts to come to the limelight from the complete darkness and Sweta Patel serving in USA, for her inspirational poem on "Dawn" for helping patients to come into the bright side from blind side with the help of a guide. Such worthy words help to harness patient's psychology positively. Science with subjective forces for health and happiness is a good idea to present.

Book editing process involves correction, condensation, orderly organization, and continuation as collaboration with the author with an intention of producing correct, consistent and complete work. It gives us immense peace and pleasure of gaining goals, which are very well supported with the editing work by Dinesh Sorani, MPT (Physical Functional Diagnosis), PhD (Physiotherapy), Senior Lecturer, Government Physiotherapy College, Jamnagar. Dr Sorani has helped us from the beginning till the end as if it is his book. Professor Dr Subhash Khatri helped us initially for the book index work. Dr Dhara Sharma of Ahmedabad Institute of Medical Science (AIMS) also helped us initially. Dr Setoo Jain, MPT (Ortho), working at AIMS college, helped in reading this book, corrections, clues and computer work. Final finishing of book work was so simple with Setoo's attentive attitude to my e-mails with receptive-responsive nature for additions and alterations.

Thanks to our past students, Dhruv Dave, Devangi Shah, Bhavesh Jagad, and Rajiv Limbasiya, for their invaluable help in preparing and presenting my PhD thesis on "Paraplegia Role Model" which is the foundation of this book.

Students are the main beneficiary of the book. Thanks to Dhara Agnihotri, MPT (Cardiopulmonary student) and Stuti Shah, MPT (Rehab student), for giving us feedback about students' need and helping us in book preparing work.

Since three years, we had an idea of presenting and pleasing our beloved students with our more than 25 years of work experience—treating patients and teaching students with SCI with rehabilitation measures. Meanwhile, I came to USA in April 2013 and other two authors and editor were in India. Thanks to the present era of technology—telephone, internet, e-mail, computers, which made our work so simple. My special thanks to my son-in-law Shri Kushal Kumar, for his gesture of giving gift of iPad and iPhone 5, which made my work of exploring-net-dictionary, text writing, e-mailing to co-authors and editor back and forth for communication and corrections.

Publishers interest to promote the thoughts of authors to the professionals is duly acknowledged. Our heart-whelming happiness is due to Shri Sharadbhai Patel of "Jaypee Brothers Medical Publishers (P) Ltd" for being instrumental in this success story.

There are two types of medical conferences—(1) Conference on medical discipline, e.g. Physiotherapy Conference and (2) Conference on conditions, e.g. International Conference on SCI. Same is true for books—some books are on subjects and some are on conditions. This book is written on spinal injury and how different professionals play roles. This book is written with the background of care and cultural systems with financial and facility status of India/Asia but many basic principles of program remains the same throughout the world, hence this book will be useful to global professionals. "A picture is worth a thousand words". With this view, we have included many relevant—real pictures of different activities of rehabilitation process and body parts.

Last but not least, to our beloved patients, relatives, and caretakers who helped us constantly and consistently by sharing their experiences, problems with us and also our students for telling us about their needs which will be of great help to the patients, partners, students and staff.

Dear readers, please read this book and heartily help the patients with spinal cord injury. Thanks and good luck!

Contents

Section 1: Information

Section 2: Investigations (Causes, Signs and Symptoms, Classifications and Investigations)

Section 3: Implementations (Management)

Part 1: Survival Stage

Section 4: Recent Research (SCI—Past, Present, Future)

Abbreviations

ADL	Activities of Daily Living
APTA	American Physical Therapy Association
ASIA	American Spinal Injury Association
ASH orthosis	Anterior Spinal Hyperextension orthosis
BBB	Blood-Brain Barrier
BMI	Body Mass Index
BCR	Bulbo Cavernosus Reflex
CPR	Cardiopulmonary Resuscitation
CSF	Cerebrospinal Fluid
COPD	Chronic Obstructive Pulmonary Disease
CT	Computerized Tomography
Conf.	Conference
DVT	Deep Vein Thrombosis
PhD	Doctor of Philosophy
EMG	Electromyography
ICD	International Classifications of Disability
KUB X-ray	Kidney Ureter Bladder X-ray
KEM	King Edward Memorial
LMNL	Lower Motor Neuron Lesion
MRI	Magnetic Resonance Imaging
MS Ortho	Master of Surgery Orthopedic
MSW	Medical Social Worker
MAS	Modified Ashworth Scale
NCV	Nerve Conduction Velocity
NGO	Non-governmental Organization
OT	Occupational Therapy

PT	Physiotherapy
P&O	Prosthetics & Orthotics
Psycho	Psychology
PFT	Pulmonary Function Test
QOL	Quality of Life
ST	Speech Therapy
SCI	Spinal Cord Injury
SOMI	Sterno-Occipital-Mandibular Immobilization
UMNL	Upper Motor Neuron Lesion
UTI	Urinary Tract Infection
WHO	World Health Organization

1
Section

Information

Chapter Outline

1. Body/Brain Structure and Systems of Functioning
2. Biomechanics of the Spine
3. Health Highlights
4. Medical Science Dimensions
5. Rehabilitation Medicine Science Dimensions

1

Body/Brain Structure and Systems of Functioning

For the management of spine and spinal cord problems in patients, it is appropriate to understand the basics of our brain and body's structure and system of their functioning. Brain cares and controls the body and body is our instrument through which we express and enjoy.

- Brain and spinal cord are body's central nervous system (CNS). Brain is the commanding center of the body and spinal cord is the conveying pathway of the messages sent from brain to body and from body to brain.
- Peripheral nervous system (PNS) is a network of nerve strands that branch off from the right and left sides of spinal cord through the openings between the each vertebra of spinal canal. These nerve pairs, spread throughout our body to deliver the commands from our brain to body parts and convey back the information.
- Muscular system moves the body parts, maintains posture and helps in blood circulations. They are of three types: 1) Skeletal, 2) Cardiac, 3) Smooth (non-striated). Skeletal muscles attached to the bones of skeletal system, are around 700 in number. They are constructed of skeletal muscle tissues, blood vessels, tendons and nerves. Muscle tissues are also found inside the heart (cardiac), digestive organ and blood vessels (smooth muscles).

BRAIN

Brain is safely secured in a hard bony covering called the skull, suspended in Cerebrospinal Fluid (CSF), isolated from blood stream by blood-brain barriers (BBB). The average weight is 1400 g (3 lb), volume 1,260 cubic centimeter in men and 1,130 cubic centimeter in women. This does not correlate in any simple way with intelligent quotient (IQ). According to the Array tomography, it is composed of 200 billion neurons, glial cells and blood vessels, 125 trillion synapses. The live Brain is very soft and pinkish gray in color.

Brain-to-body mass ratio (BMR) (Encephalization quotient) is on an average of 1:40 in humans. An overview of the brain is shown in Figures 1A to E.

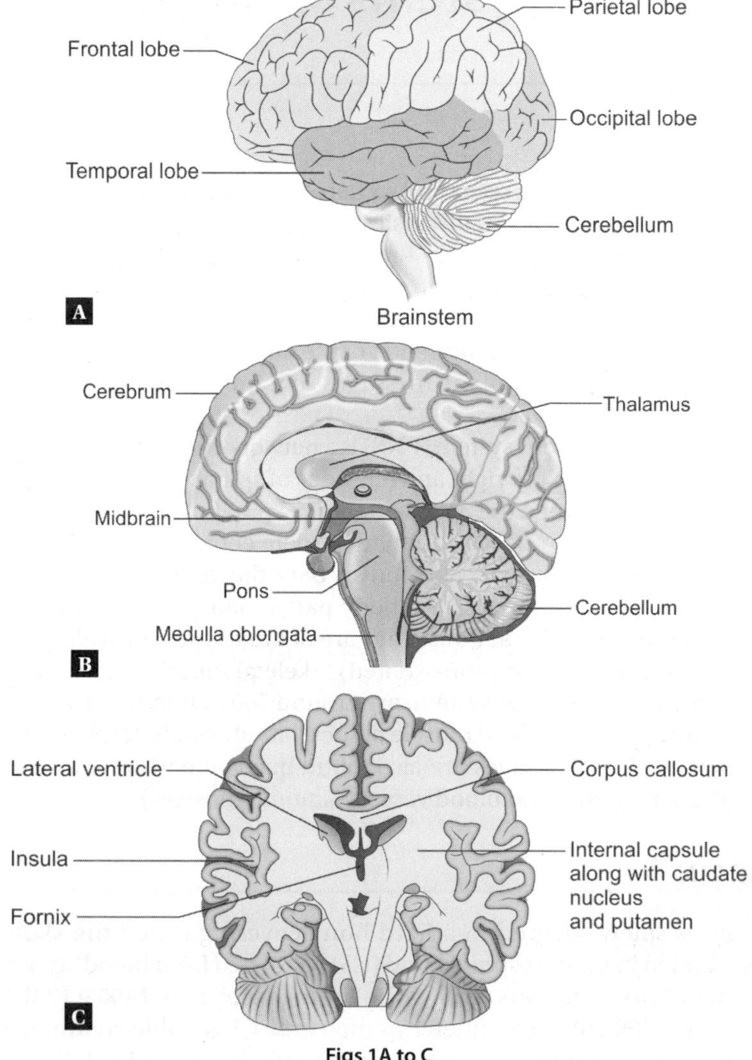

Figs 1A to C

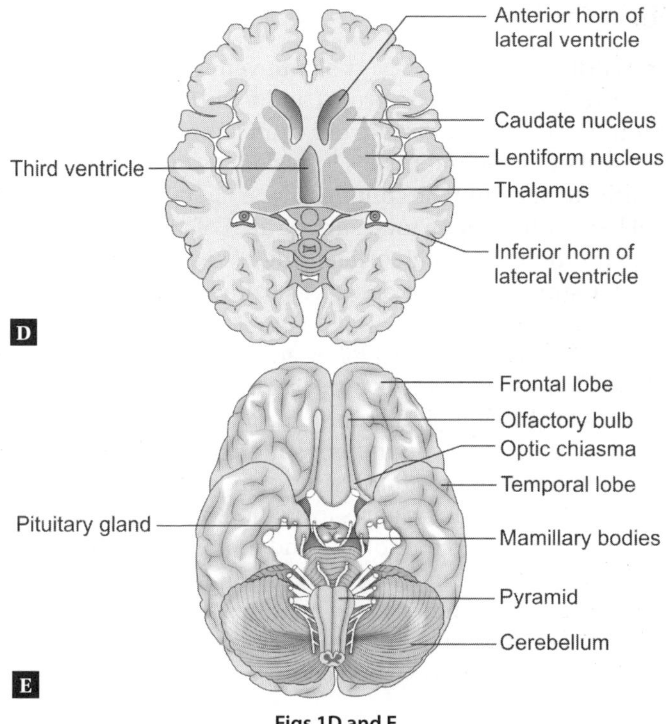

Figs 1D and E

Figs 1A to E: (A) Brain lateral view; (B) Brain midsagittal view; (C) Brain frontal section view; (D) Brain transverse section view; (E) Brain inferior view

Cerebrum

The cerebral hemispheres (cerebrum) form the largest part of the brain and are situated above other brain structures. They are covered with an outer gray matter layer, cerebral cortex which has a convoluted topography. Cerebral cortex is supported by an inner layer of white matter. Underneath the cerebrum lies the brainstem, resembling a stalk on which the cerebrum is attached. Both hemispheres communicate with each other through nerve fibers at the base of the fissure, corpus callosum and smaller commissures. At the rear of the brain, beneath the cerebrum and behind the brainstem is Cerebellum, with a horizontally furrowed surface, it looks different than any other brain parts.

Cerebral Cortex

Cerebral cortex consists of 6 layers of unmyelinated neurons (the gray matter forming cortex of cerebrum) and is situated at the top of the cerebrum. The dominant feature of a human brain is corticalization. Cortex is a sheet of neural tissues folded in a way that allows a large surface area to fit within the confines of a skull. When unfolded, each cerebral hemisphere has a total surface area of about 1.3 square feet (0.24 square meters). Each cortical ridge is called Gyrus and each groove or fissure separating one gyrus from another gyrus is called Sulcus.

The cortex is divided into 4 lobes and an additional limbic lobe. Within each lobe are numerous cortical areas. The right and left sides of the cortex are broadly similar in shape and most cortical areas are replicated on both sides. Right hemisphere controls the left side of body and left hemisphere controls the right side of body. The left is dominant in language and right is in spatiotemporal reasoning.

- Frontal lobe for problem solving and motor functions
- Parietal lobe is for sensation, body position
- Temporal lobe for memory and hearing
- Occipital lobe for visual processing
- Limbic lobe for emotional behavior.

Basal Ganglia

Basal ganglia are group of nuclei that act as a cohesive functional unit. They are situated at the base of the forebrain and are strongly connected with the cerebral cortex, thalamus and other brain areas.

Striatum—the largest component receives inputs from many brain areas but sends output only to other components of the basal ganglia.

Putamen (lateral dorsal striatum) controls motor learning, motor performance with amplitude of movement.

Caudate nucleus (medial dorsal striatum) is responsible for spatial working, memory, learning, emotions, and sleep. Damage to striatum leads to Huntington's Disease (HD) or Huntington's Chorea—a neurodegenerative genetic disorder that affects muscle coordination with abnormal involuntary jerky movements mainly at big joints. The "Athetoid" movements—slow, involuntary movement of fingers, hands, toes, arms, legs, neck, tongue (writhing movement—slow snake or worm like movement) mainly at small joints, is due to lesion in the corpus striatum.

Globus pallidus is a part of the telencephalon and a major portion of basal ganglia. It receives input from the striatum routed to thalamus and sends inhibitory output to a number of motor related areas. It has inhibitory actions that balance the excitatory actions of the cerebellum. These two systems work in harmony for the smooth and controlled movement. Imbalances can create tremors and jerks.

Substantia nigra is darker than neighboring areas located in midbrain.

- Pars compacta supplies dopamine to the striatum
- Pars reticulata conveys signals from basal ganglia to other brain structures.

Parkinson's disease—Degeneration of the dopamine producing cells in the substantia *nigra* (pars compacta) leading to "Parkinsonism disease." The symptoms of "Huntington's chorea and Parkinsonism" are opposite. Parkinson's shows gradual loss of initiation of movement where as Huntington's chorea shows inability to prevent parts from moving unintentionally. Sub-thalamic nucleus receives input mainly from striatum and cerebral cortex, and projects to the globus pallidus. Damage to this nucleus leads to "Hemiballismus" characterized by violent and uncontrollable flinging movements of arms and legs.

Internal Capsule

Internal capsule is a white matter structure which carries information past the basal ganglia. It separates caudate nucleus and thalamus from putamen and globus pallidus. It contains corticospinal tracts carrying motor information from primary motor cortex to lower motor neurons in the spinal cord. Lenticulostriate arteries supply blood to internal capsule. These small vessels are vulnerable to chronic hypertension and can result in infarction and hemiplegia.

Corpus Callosum (Tough Body)

Corpus callosum is a wide flat bundle of fibers and the largest white matter structure in the brain, consisting of 200–250 million contralateral axonal projections, situated beneath the cerebral cortex, at the longitudinal fissure. It connects both the cerebral hemispheres and facilitates inter hemispherical communications.

Midbrain

Midbrain is located below the cerebral cortex and above the hindbrain placing it at the centre of the brain. It is the smallest region of the brain that controls vision, hearing, sleep/wake, alertness and temperature. Portion of the midbrain, the red nucleus and substantia *nigra* are involved in the control of the body movement.

Brain Stem is the posterior part of the brain, continuous with the spinal cord. It includes medulla oblongata, pons and midbrain. Brainstem provides main motor and sensory supply to the face and neck through the cranial nerves. Of the twelve pairs of cranial nerves, except Ist and IInd cranial nerves, other ten pairs emerge from brainstem. It also plays an important role in regulating respiration, heart rate, and the central nervous system, maintaining consciousness, sleep cycle and eating.

Cerebellum

Cerebellum is attached to the bottom of the brain, tucked underneath the cerebral hemispheres. Its surface is covered with finely spaced parallel grooves. It does not initiate movement but with the sensory input, it produces fine motor activity, and maintains equilibrium and posture.

Thalamus

Thalamus is a midline symmetrical structure of two halves, situated between the cortex and midbrain—both in terms of location and neurological connections. Its functions are relaying sensory and motor signals to the cerebral cortex, regulating consciousness, sleep and alertness.

Hypothalamus

Hypothalamus is about a pearl or an almond size, located below the thalamus and above the midbrain. It links the nervous system with endocrine glands through the Pituitary gland. It secretes hypothalamic hormone which stimulates or inhibits the secretion of pituitary gland hormone. It controls body temperature, hunger-thirst, sleep-morning waking up, moods, sex drive, and parenting and attachment behaviors.

Pituitary Gland

Pituitary gland (Hypophysis) is the master endocrine gland, about a pea size and weighing 0.5 grams. It rests in a small bony cavity, sella turcica, covered by dural fold. It has anterior, intermediate and posterior lobes. Posterior lobe is functionally connected with hypothalamus via a small tube, called pituitary stalk. The gland secretes nine hormones that regulate homeostasis.

Ventricles

There are four cavities, two lateral ventricles, third ventricle and fourth ventricle, filled with fluid (CSF) in the middle of brain. They are interconnected. CSF is formed in ventricles by delicate tuft of tissue called choroid plexus.

Cerebrospinal Fluid

Cerebrospinal fluid (CSF) is a clear, colorless fluid, produced in the choroid plexus of the brain. CSF occupies the subarachnoid space (space between the arachnoid mater and pia mater) and the ventricular system around and inside the brain and spinal cord. It continuously circulates around the brain and the spinal cord. It cushions (or buffers) and bathes the brain and the spinal cord, within their bony confines. It provides the basic mechanical, immunological protection to brain and spinal cord. Brain floats in neutral buoyancy of CSF. It serves a vital regulation of cerebral blood flow. Our body produces 500 mL of CSF daily and it is absorbed in blood and lymphatic system. When the production and absorption balance is disrupted hydrocephalus occurs.

VERTEBRAL COLUMN

There are 33 vertebrae in the spine. Cervical 7, Thoracic 12, Lumbar 5, with 5 fused vertebrae to form Sacrum and 4 fused vertebrae to form coccyx or tail bone. The vertebrae which are not fused are separated by intervertebral discs (Fig. 2).

Vertebra

Vertebra is one of the bony or cartilaginous segments, composing the spinal column, having more or less cylindrical body, whose ends articulate by pads of cartilage with those of adjacent vertebrae and forms bony arch that encloses the spinal cord.

Intervertebral Disc

The disc lies between adjacent vertebrae in the spine. Each disc forms a cartilaginous joint to allow slight movement of the vertebrae, and acts as a ligament to hold the vertebrae together. Disc has several outer layers of fibrocartilage known as annulus fibrosus which surrounds the inner nucleus pulposus. There is a disc between each pair of vertebrae

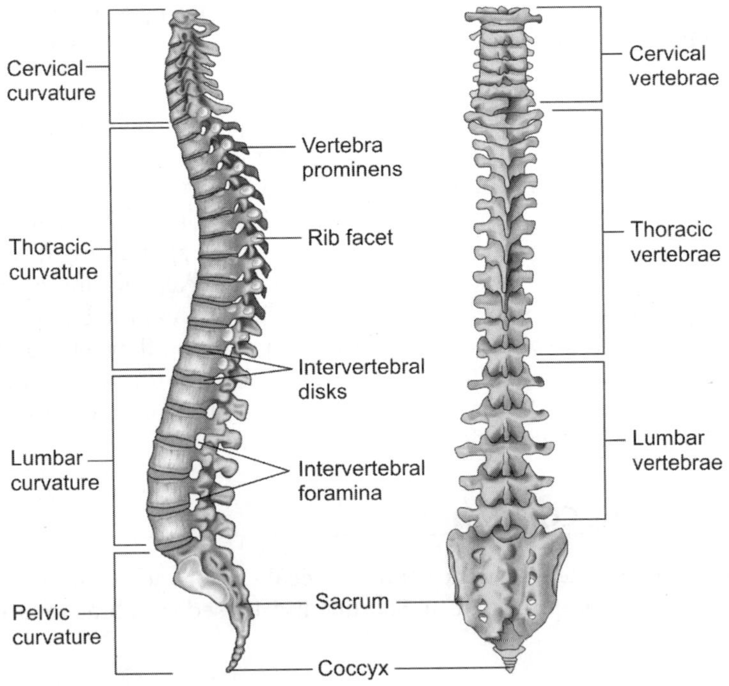

Fig. 2: Vertebral column

except for the first cervical segment, atlas and axis. There are 23 discs in human spine. The disc between cevical-5 and cervical-6 is designated as "C5-6" and similarly other discs are designated. The nucleus of disc contains mucoprotein gel which absorbs shocks and distributes weight when there is pressure. In prolapsed disc, the jelly is pushed out of disc and presses the nerve roots located near the disc, giving symptoms like Sciatica. Disc degenerates with age advancement.

Curves of Vertebral Column

- *Cervical lordosis (convex forward)* begins at the apex of the odontoid (tooth-like) process and ends at the middle of the second thoracic vertebra.
- *Thoracic kyphosis (convex backward)* begins at the middle of second and ends at middle of the 12th thoracic vertebra.
- *Lumbar lordosis (convex forward)* is more marked in female than in male. It begins at the middle of the last thoracic vertebra and ends at sacrovertebral angle.
- *Pelvic curve (convexity backward and downward)* begins at the sacrovertebral articulation and ends at point of the coccyx.

The trunk along with the spine provide, platform and constantly backs up the functioning of head and neck, both upper and lower extremities.

SPINAL CORD

The brain and spinal cord together, make up the central nervous system (CNS). The enclosing bony vertebral column protects the spinal cord. It is a long thin ovoid-shaped, tubular bundle of nervous tissues and support cells. In cross-section, the mantle layer develops a characteristic "butterfly" shape of gray matter. The cord begins at foramen magnum of the occipital bone (Medulla oblongata) and extends down to the space between the first and second lumbar vertebra (Conus medullaris terminates in a fibrous extension known as the Filum terminale). It doesn't extend the entire length of vertebral column. At the time of birth, the length of cord and vertebral column is equal but afterwards the vertebral column outgrows the cord. On an average in an adult, it is 45 cm (18 inches) long in men and 43 cm (17 inches) long in women. The cord has varying width ranging from 1/2 inch in cervical and lumbar to 1/4 inch thick in thoracic area. The cord is protected by three layers—Dura mater, Arachnoid mater, Pia mater of meninges and further protected by bony vertebral column.

- Dura mater is the outermost and it forms a tough protective coating. Between the dura mater and the surrounding bone of the vertebra is a space called the Epidural space. It is filled with adipose (fat) tissue, and it contains a network of blood vessels
- Arachnoid mater is the middle protective layer. It has a spider-web like appearance. The space between the arachnoid and the underlying pia mater is called the subarachnoid space. This space contains CSF. The medical procedure known as the Lumbar puncture involves use of a needle to withdraw CSF from the subarachnoid space, usually from the lumbar region
- Pia mater is the innermost protective layer. It is very delicate and it is tightly associated with the surface of the spinal cord. The cord is stabilized within the dura mater by the connecting denticulate ligaments. The dural sac ends at the vertebral level of the second sacral vertebra.

In cross-section, the peripheral region of the cord contains neural white mater tract containing sensory and motor neurons. Internal to this peripheral region is the gray butterfly-shaped central region made up of nerve cells bodies (Anterior horn cells contains motor cells whereas posterior horn contains sensory cells). This central region surrounds the central canal, which is an anatomic extension of spaces in the brain known as ventricles and, like the ventricles it contains CSF.

Emerging Nerve Pairs

- 07 cervical segments forming 08 pairs of cervical nerves
- 12 thoracic segments forming 12 pairs of thoracic nerves
- 05 lumbar segments forming 05 pairs of lumbar nerves
- 05 sacral segments forming 05 pairs of sacral nerves
- 04 coccygeal segments joined up to become single segment forming 1 pair of coccygeal nerve.

There is a discrepancy in cord and vertebral column. The cord is shorter than the vertebral column. To determine the spinal segment, following is the formula:

- Add 1 to cervical vertebra
- Add 2 to thoracic vertebra T1 to T6
- Add 3 to thoracic vertebra T7 to T9
- L1 and L2 spinal segments lie at the level of 10th thoracic vertebra
- L3 and L4 spinal segments lie at the level of 11th thoracic vertebra

- L5 spinal segment lie at the 12th thoracic vertebra
- Sacral and coccygeal segments lie at the level of L1 vertebra.

Blood

Blood to the cord is supplied by the three longitudinal arteries (Fig. 3):

- Anterior spinal artery
- Right posterior spinal artery
- Left posterior spinal artery.

They travel in the subarachnoid space and send branches into the spinal cord. Segmental medullary arteries form anastomoses (connections) with the anterior and posterior spinal arteries. They enter the spinal cord at various points along with its length.

The major contribution to the arterial blood supply of the spinal cord below the cervical region is from the radially arranged posterior and anterior radicular arteries. The largest of the anterior radicular arteries is known as anterior radicular magma (ARM) which arises between L1-2 but can arise anywhere from T9 to L5.

Ligaments (Fig. 4)

Ligaments are fibrous bands of connective tissues, strong but stretchable, provide a natural brace along with tendons and muscles, to help protect the spine from hyperflexion, hyperextension or rotational injuries. They aid stability at rest and allow guarded mobility.

- *Anterior longitudinal ligament (ALL)*—a Primary spine stabilizer, about an inch wide, runs the entire length of spine from the base of

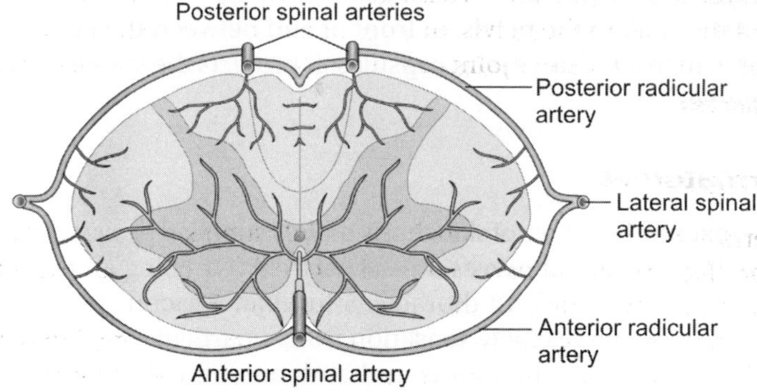

Fig. 3: Spinal cord blood supply

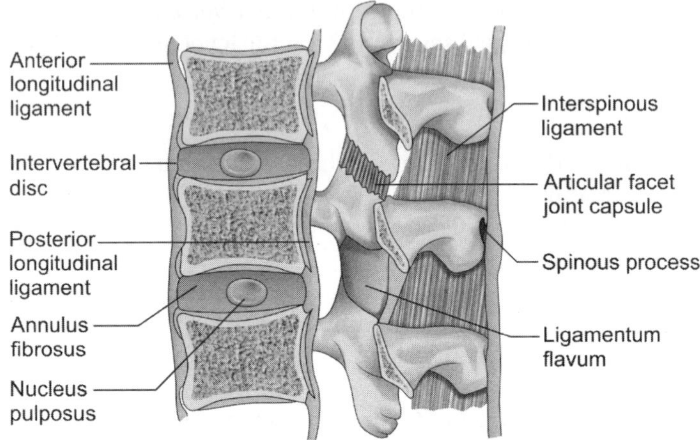

Fig. 4: Ligaments of spinal cord (Lumbar Region)

the skull to the sacrum. It connects the front (anterior) of vertebral body to the front of annulus fibrosis

- *Posterior longitudinal ligament (PLL)*—a Primary spine stabilizer, about one inch wide, runs the entire length of spine from base of the skull to the sacrum. It connects the back (posterior) of vertebral body to the back of annulus fibrosis
- *Supraspinous ligament*—Attaches the tip of each spinous process to other
- *Interspinous ligament*—A thin ligament attaches to another ligament called Ligamentum flavum that runs deep into the spinal column
- *Ligamentum flavum*—A strongest yellow ligament runs from base of the skull to the pelvis, in front of and between the lamina and also in front of facet joint capsules. It protects the spinal cord and nerves.

Dermatomes

A dermatome is an area of skin that is mainly supplied by a single spinal nerve (Fig. 5). Spinal nerves are—8 cervical (C1 being an exception with no dermatome), 12 thoracic, 5 lumbar, 5 sacral, 1 coccygeal. Each of these nerves relay sensation from a particular region of skin to the brain. Along the thorax and abdomen, the dermatomes are like a stack of disc forming human, each supplied by different spinal

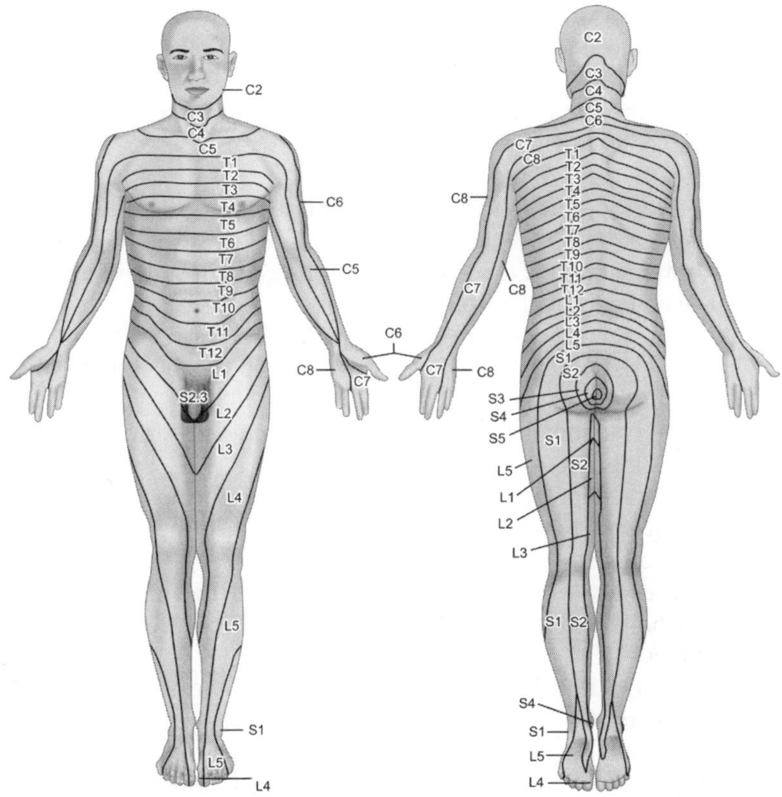

Fig. 5: Dermatomes

nerve. In the legs and arms, the pattern is different; the dermatomes run longitudinally along the limbs. Although, the general pattern is similar in all people, the precise areas of innervation are as unique to an individual as finger prints.

Dermatomes and Anatomical Landmarks

- C2—1 cm lateral to the occipital protuberance at the base of skull, behind the ear
- C3—In the supraclavicular fossa at the midclavicular line
- C4—Over the acromioclavicular joint
- C5—On the radial side of antecubital fossa, just proximal to the elbow joint
- C6—On the dorsal surface of the proximal phalanx of the thumb

- C7—On the dorsal surface of the proximal phalanx of middle finger
- C8—On the dorsal surface of the proximal phalanx of the little finger
- T1—On the ulnar side of the antecubital fossa, proximal to the medial epicondyle of the humerus
- T2—At the apex of the axilla
- T3—Intersection of the midclavicular line and the 3rd intercostal space
- T4—Intersection of the midclavicular line and the 4th intercostal space at the level of nipple
- T5—Intersection of the midclavicular line and the 5th intercostal space horizontally located midway between the level of nipples and xiphoid process
- T6—Intersection of the midclavicular line and the horizontal level of xiphoid process
- T7—Intersection of the midclavicular line and the horizontal level at one quarter the distance between the level of of xiphoid process and umbilicus
- T8—Intersection of the midclavicular line and the horizontal level at one half the distance between the level of xiphoid process and umbilicus
- T9—Intersection of the midclavicular line and the horizontal level at three quarter the distance between the level of xiphoid process and umbilicus
- T10—Intersection of the midclavicular line, at the horizontal level of umbilicus
- T11—Intersection of the midclavicular line, at the horizontal level midway between the level of umbilicus and inguinal ligament
- T12—Intersection of the midclavicular line and the midpoint of inguinal ligament
- L1—Midway between the key sensory points for T12 and L2
- L2—On the anterior medial thigh, at the midpoint of a line connecting the midpoint of the inguinal ligament and the medial epicondyle of the femur
- L3—At the medial epicondyle of the femur
- L4—Over the medial malleolus
- L5—On the dorsum of the foot at the 3rd metatarsophalangeal joint
- S1—On the lateral aspects of the calcaneus
- S2—At the midpoint of the popliteal fossa

- S3—Over the tuberosity of ischium or infragluteal fold
- S4–S5—In the perineal area, less than one cm, lateral to the mucocutaneous zone.

Myotomes

Myotomes' testing is an integral part of neurological examination as each nerve root coming from the spinal cord supplies the specific group of muscles. Testing of the myotome, in the form of isometric resisted muscle testing, provides the clinician with information about the level in spine where a lesion may be present. Results may indicate the lesion to spinal cord nerve root, or intervertebral disc herniation pressing on the spinal nerve roots.

Myotomes distribution of upper and lower limbs:

Upper extremity	*Lower extremity*
C1-2 Neck flexion/extension	L2 Hip flexion
C3 Neck lateral flexion	L3 Knee extension
C4 Shoulder elevation	L4 Ankle dorsiflexion
C5 Shoulder abduction	L5 Great toe extension
C6 Elbow flexion/Wrist extension	S1 Ankle plantar flexion
C7 Elbow extension/Wrist flexion	S2 Knee flexion
C8 Thumb extension	
T1 Finger abduction	

Difference between the Dermatomes and Myotomes: Myotome is the group of muscles that a single nerve root innervates, whereas Dermatome is an area of skin that a single nerve root innervates.

Tendons

Tendons consist of densely packed collagen fibers, similar to ligament except these tension—withstanding fibrous tissues attach muscles to the bone.

Muscular System

Muscular system of the spine is very complex. They are in superficial and deep layers. Muscles, individually or in groups, are supported by fascia. Fascia is a strong sheath-like connective tissue. The tendon that attaches the muscle to bone is part of the fascia.

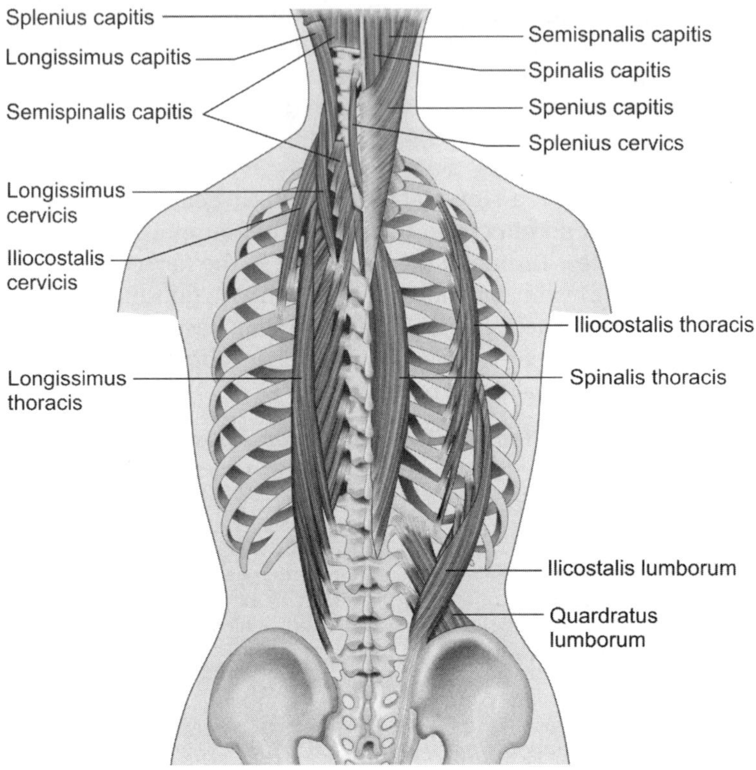

Fig. 6: Muscles vertebral column (deep layer)

Muscles of the Posterior Cervical and Thoracic Spine (Deep Layer) (Fig. 6)

- Semispinalis Capitis—Head rotation/pulls backwards
- Iliocostalis Cervicis—Extends cervical vertebrae
- Longissimus Cervicis—Extends cervical vertebrae
- Longissimus Capitis—Head rotation/pulls backwards
- Longissimus Thoracis—Extension/lateral flexion of vertebral column; rib rotation
- Iliocostalis Thoracis—Extension/lateral flexion of vertebral column; rib rotation
- Semispinalis Thoracis—Extends and rotates vertebral column
- Sternocleidomastoid—Head flexion, side flexion same side, rotation to opposite.

Muscles of the Lumbar Region

- Psoas major—Flexes the thigh at hip joint and vertebral column
- Quadratus lumborum—Lateral flexion of the vertebral column
- Multifidus—Fixing of one vertebra with adjoining vertebra; extension and rotation.

Muscles of the Back and Front (Superficial Layer)

There are many muscles on the front and back side of the trunk, prime purpose is to maintain the posture and provide platform for the motions of head and limbs.

Spine Functions (Vertebral Column)

- Protects spinal cord and nerve roots, also protects internal organs
- Provides base for attachments to muscles, ligaments, tendons
- Provides structural support to head, neck and chest
- Connects upper and lower body segments
- Maintains the balance and weight distribution of body
- Provides flexibility and mobility
- Other functions—Red blood cell production, mineral storage.

Importance of "S" Shape Curve of Spine

- "S" curve and intervertebral discs absorb the shocks
- Meets the problems of the weight of the visceral organs
- Provides additional space for viscera
- Weight distribution of entire body: Cervical curve—the head; Thoracic curve—the chest organs; Lumbar curve—the pelvic organs
- The curvature with vertebral fragments and springy arrangement protects vertebral column from breakage
- Provides aesthetic look to our posture, motion and gait.

Spinal Cord Functions

Spinal cord is the informative highway between the brain and rest of the body. Ascending tracts carry information (feeding brain) from body, and the descending tracts convey commands from brain to body (Fig 7).

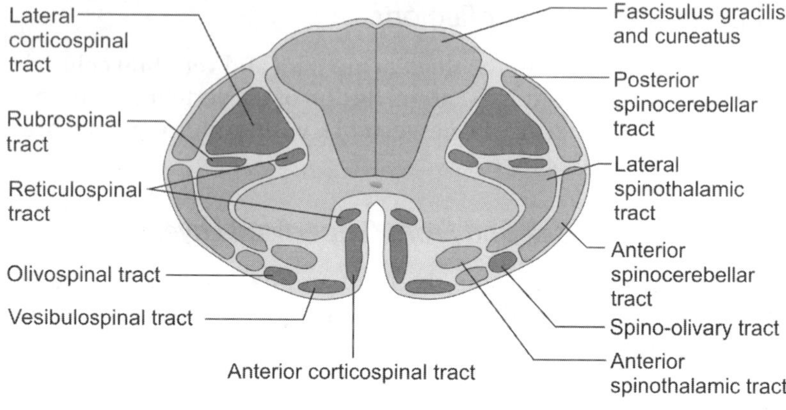

Fig. 7: Tracts of spinal cord

- Somatosensory organization—a) Dorsal column medial lemniscus tract (touch, proprioception, vibratory sensory pathway). b) anterolateral system ALS (pain, temperature sensory pathway)
- Motor organization—The corticospinal tract (Pyramidal tracts) serves as the motor pathway for upper motor neuronal signals, coming from cerebral cortex and from primitive brainstem motor nuclei going down towards body parts.

PERIPHERAL NERVOUS SYSTEM

Peripheral nervous system (PNS) consists of nerves and ganglions outside the brain and the spinal cord. The main function of the PNS is to serve as a communication relay connecting the brain with body. Unlike CNS, the PNS is not protected by skull, spinal bones or blood-brain barrier, leaving it exposed to toxins and injuries. It is divided into somatic nervous system, autonomic nervous system and sensory nervous system (Fig. 8).

Cranial Nerves

There are 12 pairs of cranial nerves and are a part of PNS with an exception of second cranial nerve (optic nerve) (Table 1).

Neuromuscular junction connects the nervous system to muscular system via synapses between the efferent nerve fiber and muscle fiber.

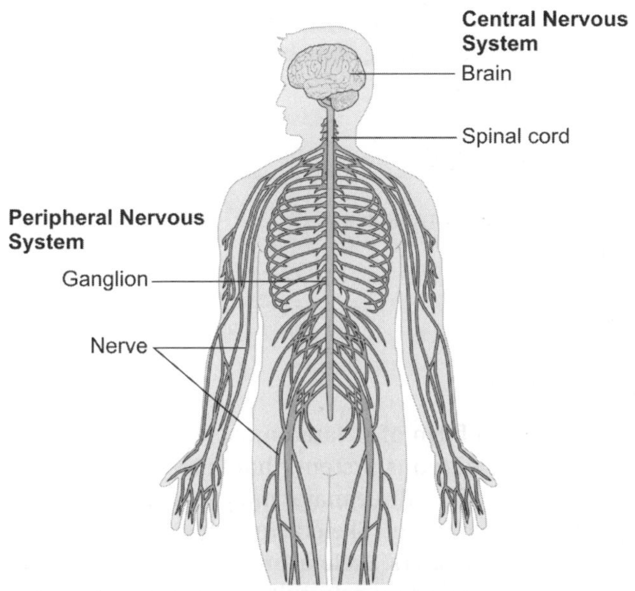

Fig. 8: Peripheral nervous system

Table 1: 12 pairs of cranial nerves

No.	*Cranial nerve*	*Major function*
I	Olfactory	Smell
II	Optic	Vision
III	Oculomotor	Eyelid and eyeball movement
IV	Trochlear	Turns eye downward and inward
V	Trigeminal	Chewing, face and mouth-touch and pain
VI	Abducens	Turns eye laterally
VII	Facial	Facial expressions, secretes saliva, tears and taste
VIII	Vestibulocochlear	Hearing, equilibrium (Auditory)
IX	Glossopharangeal	Taste, senses carotid blood pressure
X	Vagus	Senses aortic blood pressure, slows heart rate, stimulates digestive organs, taste
XI	Spinal accessory	Trapezius, sternocleidomastoid, swallowing movement
XII	Hypoglossal	Tongue movement

Motor neurons release the acetylcholine (ACh), a small molecule neurotransmitter. The binding of ACh to the receptor can depolarize the muscle fiber to contract.

MUSCULAR SYSTEM

There are three types of muscles:

1. Skeletal.
2. Smooth.
3. Cardiac.

Skeletal Muscle

Skeletal muscle is a form of striated muscle tissue which is under control of somatic nervous system, that is to say, it is voluntarily controlled. It is one of the three major muscle types, the others being cardiac and smooth muscles. Skeletal muscles are attached to bones by bundles of collagen fibers. Skeletal muscle is made up of individual component, myocytes or muscle cells or muscle fibers. These log cylindrical multinucleated cells are also called myofibers. Myofibers are in turn composed of myofibrils. Myofibrils are composed of actin and myosin units in sarcomere, the basic functional unit of a muscle. The actin filaments slide past the myosin filaments toward the middle of the sarcomere. The result is the shortening of the sarcomere. The term muscle refers to multiple bundles of muscle fibers held together by connective tissues. Muscle fibers have capability to contract and relax.

Smooth Muscle

Smooth muscles are involuntary nonstriated muscles, divided into single unit and multiunits. A substantial portion of the cytoplasm of smooth muscle cells is taken up by the molecules Actin and Myosin, which together have the capability to contract. Smooth muscle fibers have a fusiform shape and like striated muscle can become tense and relax. They demonstrate greater elasticity and function within a larger length tension curve than striated muscle. This ability to stretch and still maintain contractibility is important in organs like the intestine and urinary bladder. In the relaxed state, each cell is spindle-shaped 20–500 micrometers in length. Smooth muscles are found within the walls of blood vessels, tunica media layer of large (aorta) and small arteries, arterioles, veins, lymphatic vessels, urinary bladder, uterus, male and female reproductive tracts, gastrointestinal tract, respiratory tract, pili of skin, the ciliary muscle, glomeruli of kidney and iris of the eye. Smooth muscle is fundamentally different from skeletal muscle and cardiac muscle in terms of structure, function, regulation of contraction and excitation-contraction coupling. Single unit variety—either the whole muscle contract or whole muscle relax.

Cardiac Muscle

Cardiac muscle is a type of involuntary striated muscle found in the walls of and histological foundation of the heart, especially myocardium. The cell cardiomyocytes contain only one unique nucleus. Cardiac muscle exhibit cross striations formed by alternating segments of thick and thin protein filaments. Like skeletal muscle, the primary structural proteins of cardiac muscle are Actin (thin-lighter appearance) and Myosin (thick-darker appearance). Coordinated contractions of cardiac muscle cell in the heart push the blood out of atria and ventricle. Cardiac muscle like all tissues in the body, rely on an ample blood supply, through coronary artery. In contrast to skeletal muscle, cardiac muscle requires extracellular calcium ions for contraction to occur.

2

Biomechanics of the Spine

BIOMECHANICS

Mechanics is the study of the interactions between matter and the force acting on it. It is divided into i) Static, ii) Dynamic, iii) Kinematics.

Static means no change in momentum while dynamic deals with force and why objects move. Kinematics is the description of how objects move. Kinematics is the study (calculating velocity, acceleration, etc.) of the state of motion of a body without taking into account the cause of force. It includes both resting and moving bodies. Kinetics is the study of moving bodies only in relation with force or torque.

Flexion, extension, lateral flexion and rotations are available motions at the spine. At individual level these motions are coupled. Coupling is defined as the consistent association of one motion about an axis to another motion around a different axis. Pure lateral flexion and rotation doesn't occur in any portion of the spine. Coupling pattern as well as the type and amount of motions that are available are complex. It differs from region to region and depends on the spinal posture, curve orientation of facet, fluidity, elasticity and thickness of intervertebral disc. Motions at interbody and facet joints are interdependent. Amount of motion=size of disc. Direction of motion= facet joint orientation. The intervertebral disc increases range of motion and in its absence only translation occurs. The nucleus pulposus behaves like fluid. Both annulus fibrosus and nucleus pulposus help in achieving tremendous amount of range of motion at spine. But the facet orientation acts on direction of the motion, e.g. If superior and inferior facets of the three adjacent vertebrae is in frontal plane then lateral flexion and rotation will be more. On the other hand, if it is in sagittal plane then flexion and extension is facilitated. Facet in upper thoracic region is more in frontal plane so flexion and extension is limited and in lower thoracic and lumbar region it is more in sagittal plane so flexion and extension is more.

Flexion

In vertebral flexion, anterior tilting and gliding of the superior vertebra occurs and causes widening of the intervertebral foramen and separation of spinous process. Amount of tilting depends upon—size of the disc, tension in supraspinous and interspinous ligaments, passive tension in facet joint capsule- Ligamentum flavum, posterior longitudinal ligament, posterior annulus fibrous. Back extension muscles work to control flexion. Annulus fibrosus compresses anteriorly and get bulged whereas posterior portion is stretched and resists separation of vertebral bodies.

Extension

The superior vertebra tilts posteriorly and glides on the inferior vertebra and causes narrowing of intervertebral foramen and the spinous process moves close together in extension. Amount of motion is limited by—bony contact of spinous process, size of the disc, passive tension in facet joint capsule, anterior longitudinal ligament, anterior trunk muscles, and anterior fibers of annulus fibrosus. The ligamentous limit to flexion is more than extension. Only anterior longitudinal ligament limits extension may be because of this reason it is very strong.

Lateral Flexion

In lateral flexion, the superior vertebra laterally tilts, rotates and translates over the adjacent vertebra below. The annulus fibrosus is compressed on the side of concavity of the curve and is stretched on the convexity of the curve. The direction of the rotation that accompanies lateral flexion differs slightly from region to region because of the orientation of the facet joints. Limits to lateral flexion are intertransverse ligaments, passive tension in annulus fibrosus and passive tension in anterior and posterior muscles on the side of the convexity.

Torsion

Torsion forces occur in axial rotation as a part of coupling. The torsion force in flexion and lateral flexion, in the lower thoracic and lumbar region is more than the upper thoracic region. It is due to the anatomical structure of the outer layer of intervertebral disc, facet orientation and vertebral bodies. When the disc is subjected to torsion, half of the fibers of annulus fibrosus resist clockwise rotation and other half resist counter clockwise rotation. But if the high amount of torsional force, bending and axial loading is combined, rupture of the disc takes place early and easily.

Shear

The force which causes sliding from side to side and from anterior to posterior is the shear force. It acts in between the disc and the vertebra causing the movement of the vertebra. The excessive shearing force can cause excessive anterior or posterior translation of one vertebra on another vertebra resulting in either subluxation or dislocation. The excessive force is resisted by facet joint locking and the disc but if there is excessive sustained load then the disc exhibits creep and facet joint resists the motion.

Core Stability

Core (central) stability is to tone up and tune up the muscles around navel/umbilicus to gain and maintain stability around the body's center of gravity.

Center of Gravity (COG): In the anatomical standing position, the COG is near navel/umbilicus, anterior to the second sacral vertebra.

Line of Gravity (LOG): In an anatomical standing position, often seen as plumb line, when viewed from side, it passes near ear canal, top of the head of the humerus, top of the head of femur, slightly behind the middle of knee, middle of the lateral malleolus.

Pelvic Tilt

It is the orientation of the pelvis in respect to femur in space:

- *Anterior pelvic tilt*—The anterior superior iliac spines (ASIS) drop forward due to short hip flexors, weak abdominals, and big belly with lengthened hip extensors. There is increased lumbar lordosis. Strengthening of lower abdominal will reduce the tilt

- *Posterior pelvic tilt*—The anterior superior iliac spines go up due to lengthened hip flexors and shortened gluteus maximus. The lumbar lordosis is flattened
- *Lateral pelvic tilt*—Left or right tilting of spine due to scoliosis of spine, short one limb, and hip or knee flexor tightness/contracture, one side weak hip abductors.

Core stability is to provide stable central part of the body for balance and for desired body movements. It involves the abdominal wall, pelvis, lower back and the diaphragm. The muscles are: 1) Multifidus—a muscle which connects the two adjoining vertebra (This muscle needs repeated recruitment and activation to hold the two vertebra in an alignment), 2) Erector spinae—holds the spine erect, 3) Transverse abdominis, 4) Internal and External obliques, 5) Quadratus lumborum, 6) Diaphragm (Breathing varies for core stability in moving and lifting), 7) Pelvic floor muscles, 8) Lumbar spine muscles, 9) Hip muscles.Before any movement or lifting, the core region is tensed first. Core stability is essential for the upright posture, motion and lifting. Without core stability, the lower back is unsupported from inside and can cause lower back pain, poor posture and lethargy.

PATHOMECHANICS

Cervical Spine

Disc pain occurs due to sustained axial load and other force like shear and torsion and as a result the degenerative changes start taking place in the disc. Moreover, the incorrect posture like forward head causes excessive flexion load on the lower cervical spine causing disc degeneration. In cervical spine, there is no posterolateral annulus fibrosus (Lind B et al. Range of motion the cervical spine. Arch Phys Medi Rehab. 1989).

The pain may be possible from the strain or tear of the anterior annulus fibrosus, especially following hyperextension trauma and strain the lateral portion of the posterior longitudinal ligament by a disc bulge (Mercer SR et al. The ligament and annulus fibrosus of human adult cervical intervertebral disc spine.1999; 24:619-26).

The facet joint gets maximum load when the cervical spine is in extension. Repetitive overwork of the facet joint and loading of the joint can result in facet joint arthropathy.

The cervical spine injury occurs most in accidents causing whiplash injury. In the whiplash injury, there is hyperextension of the cervical spine which cause cord trauma. Even if the head gets steady by colliding with the steering wheel, the inertia of the trunk will cause the hyperextensive force at the cervical spine, causing cord trauma and trauma of the surrounding ligaments, muscles of the cervical spine. The cervical spine in neutral has an extension curve, i.e. normal cervical lordosis. But when the cervical spine is flexed to 30 degree, it becomes straight like segment; if in this state excessive axial loading occurs (while gardening, something hits the head from above). It can cause injury of the cervical spine along with cord.

Trauma in players: Cervical spine injury is common in football players, wrestlers and gymnastics. Football players, wearing helmet, try to hit ball with head will cause shearing force. In shearing, the axial load and compressive load increases beyond the limits of cervical spine resulting in the injury of the cervical spine and the cord.

Thoracic Spine

The pathomechanics of the thoracic spine remains same as that of the cervical spine. In the thoracic spine, the LOG falls in front of the thoracic vertebra. This causes forward flexion posture of the thoracic spine and so there is Kyphosis. In normal biomechanics, the flexed position and flexion movement of the thoracic spine is checked and controlled by the extensors and the posterior ligaments of the thoracic spine.

If the head and neck remains more in flexion due to work, it will further increase the kyphosis, vice-a-versa or if the flexion movement of the thoracic is increased, it will keep the head and neck in forward position, this will also cause more kyphosis of the thoracic spine.

If there is excessive compressive force on the straight spine, it will cause *burst fracture* of the vertebra. But if there is excessive compressive force on relatively flexed thoracic spine, it will cause *wedge fracture* of the vertebra. In osteoporosis and with muscular weakness, the thoracic spine will be more in flexion than normal kyphosis. In this situation, if there is more loading on the anterior part of the vertebra and with the weak osteoporotic vertebral bones, it will cause *wedge fracture* of the vertebra.

Lumbar Spine

The compressive loads causing fracture in lumbar spine is very common in osteoporotic patients. The epiphyseal ring of the lumbar spine is very prone to the development of abnormal ossification which can result in epiphysitis or Scheuermann's disease.

The vascularity of the lumbar is good, so it helps in early healing of the fractures but it can also cause spread of metastatic lesions of surrounding structures into lumbar vertebra.

It is believed that the capsule of the facet joint of lumbar spine is having meniscoid inclusions, if some jerky movements occur like sudden flexion or extension, then there are chances that these meniscoid inclusions can get entrapped into joint itself giving immense pain of sudden onset.

The annulus fibrosus gets compressed on the side of side bending and gets subjected to the tensile force on opposite side (White and Punjabi).

If hamstrings are tight, they alter the lumbopelvic rhythm by restricting the forward rotation of the pelvis in standing; this causes compensation from lumbar, i.e. excessive lumbar flexion which can cause damage to the posterior structure of the lumbar spine. Thus, resulting in low back pain. A slow casual walk reduces spine motion and produces static loading of the tissues whereas fast walking with arms swinging causes cycling loading of the tissues. Thus, due to cycling loading certain patients have relief from back pain during walking.

Forward bending with neutral lumbar spine helps the extensor muscles to oppose the anterior forces and the force of gravity which acts on lumbar vertebra, thus prevents the structure from getting injured. But if the lumbar spine is flexed while lifting or bending forward then the orientation of the muscle action gets changed thus they can't oppose the shear forces and gravity force acting on the lumbar vertebra thus sometimes causing damage to the vertebra.

3

Health Highlights

The word health is derived from an English word “hoelth” meaning being sound—a state of complete Physical, Mental, Social well-being and not mere absence of disease or infirmity (WHO-1946 New York). The other factors included are vocational (economic) and spirituality for a sound health (Fig. 1).

BODY MASS INDEX

Body mass index (BMI) is a number calculated from a person’s height and weight. BMI provides a reliable indicator for body fatness for

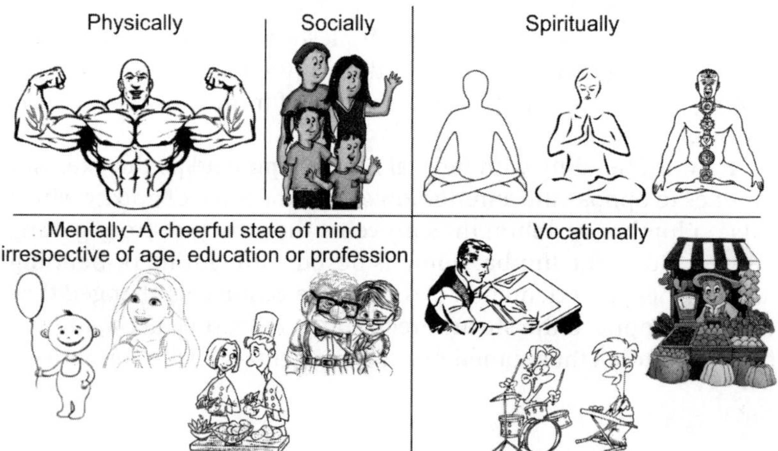

Fig. 1: Different aspects of health

most people and is used to screen weight categories that are prone to health problems.

$$BMI = \frac{Mass\ or\ Weight\ (Kg)}{[Height(m)]^2}$$

No.	Category	BMI (adult)
1	Under weight	18.5 and below
2	Normal Healthy weight	18.5 to 24.9
3	Over weight	25.0 to 29.9
4	Obese	30.0 and above

4

Medical Science Dimensions

INTRODUCTION

Medical science has following three dimensions:
- Preventive medicine
- Curative medicine
- Rehabilitation medicine.

Preventive Medicine

Preventive medicine or preventive healthcare or prophylaxis measures, consists of taking measures to prevent the disease or damage (injury) rather than curing or treating their symptoms. The preventive medicine with public health methods which works at the level of population health and curative medicine works at individual health.

- *Primary prevention:* Methods to avoid occurrence of disease (Population and community-based health promotions)
  - Vaccination: Polio, Smallpox, Tuberculosis, Measles, Mumps, Influenza, etc. Mass vaccination in a particular province, provides eradication of the viruses from that province and the disease (e.g. Pulse polio program)
  - Sanitation: Clean surroundings
  - Hygiene: Personal—Body bath, hand washing, clean clothes
  - Intake: Clean air, water, food
  - Nutritive diet: Balanced (amount and ingredients) nutritive diet with timings
  - Habits: Balance between activities and rest with a sound sleep
  - Bad habits: Avoid smoking, alcohol, narcotic drugs
  - Mind control over anger, quarreling

    - Regular exercises and practising pranayama and yoga to keep the body and brain fit and fine
    - Occupational hazards: Safety steps to avoid occupational injuries (e.g. safety harnessing belt for a worker on electric pole to avoid fall and SCI)
    - Traffic rules observance to prevent accidental injuries
    - Polypill for prevention of disease, e.g. cardiovascular diseases
    - Education about potent threat to health.
- *Secondary prevention:* Method to diagnose the existing disease at an early stage and to do early intervention, e.g. cerebral palsy
- *Tertiary prevention:* Methods to reduce negative impact of the existing disease on functions and to reduce disease related complications.

Curative Medicine and Palliative Care

It is a healthcare discipline, oriented towards seeking cure of the existing disease. Palliative care concentrates on reducing the severity of the disease symptoms, e.g. pain.

Rehabilitation Medicine

'Re' means 'again'. Rehabilitation is a general term used to help reach to a former state of health or life and living in surroundings. After the natural or man-made disaster, there is widespread loss. There is a personal loss to the human body, there is infrastructure damage, e.g. houses, shops, schools, roads, drainage, food and water supply, electricity, communication network, TV and entertainment gadgets.

Rehabilitation process in general, is the restoration of infrastructure with restoration of disabled person's functions and to bring back that damaged province to a previous or worth living situation.

Rehabilitation medicine is a combined and coordinated team work of patient, family and friends, medical, physical medicine, social, NGO and the efforts to reach the highest possible level of functional ability to lead a quality of life (QoL) for a disabled person to the physical, mental, vocational, social and spiritual well-being. Once the recovery and restoration has reached to plateau, the disabled/differently-abled person is taught and trained to maximize with the abilities and disabilities and to retrain the person to "return to living" and to involve, integrate the person in the family, society and to the work place by rehabilitation medicine.

This branch uses the available Rehab-medicine resources to reduce and limit the impairments and disabilities, maximize the person's potential, minimize the sufferings and promote the person's adjustments with the irremediable conditions, back to the previous state of living or a meaningful living with an altered lifestyle.

HISTORY OF PHYSICAL AND REHABILITATION MEDICINE

All the professions have evolved from the primitive functioning. A "Dai" who used to do delivery is now done by the gynecologist. "Bone-setters" who were treating fracture is now done by the Orthopedic surgeon. "Munim" who maintained account is now done by Chartered Accountant. Physiotherapy (PT) has also evolved from primitive functioning. Physical means for healing have been in practice since the prehistoric time. Since the beginning of time, people have used physical agents for healing like water, heat, cold, soft tissue manipulations, exercises, heliotherapy (sun rays). Written accounts of use of physical techniques for healing can be traced as far back as the writings of Hippocrates in 460 BC. After development of orthopedics in 18th century, gymnastic was developed to treat the disabling condition, later it was known as Physiotherapy.

The Swedish word "physical therapy" means the one who is involved in gymnastics for those who are ill. In 1813, Ling founded "Royal Central Institute of Gymnastics". In 1887, PTs were given registration by Sweden's National Board of Health and Welfare. In 1894, four nurses in UK formed "Chartered Society of Physiotherapy". Schools of Physiotherapy were started in 1913 in New Zealand, in 1918 at Reed's Army Hospital in Washington DC. The first OT school was established at KEM Hospital, Mumbai in 1951, with the efforts of Kamala Nimbkar. The first PT school was started with the help of WHO in 1952 at KEM Hospital, Mumbai. In 1921, American Physical Therapy Association (APTA) was established. In 1953, Indian Association of Physiotherapy was established.

It was not until after World War I and II, to understand the necessity for more advanced treatment and rehabilitation for disabled. The public become more aware of the rehabilitation efforts due to the substantial numbers of debilitating war injuries plus the thousands of individuals disabled by a poliomyelitis epidemic. The realization of polio in the person of US President Franklin D Roosevelt, who had regained his capacity to return to public life after physical therapy at Georgia Warm Springs, USA.

The education in physical therapy started in the form of 3 months training program to 1 year program, to a 2 years diploma then the 3 years degree to 3 years plus 6 months internship to a present 4 years and 6 months of internship. Bachelor and Master in physical therapy, Doctorate in physical therapy and PhD in physical therapy are the present era programs.

Philosophy of Rehabilitation Medicine

"Self with Ethical aspects and Human rights"

Access to rehabilitation is a basic human right guaranteed by: (1) United Nations (1993); (2) European year for people with disability (2003); (3) 58th resolution of World Health Assembly (2005); (4) Persons with disability Act PWD, India (1995); (5) Many nations have anti-discriminative legislation.

The use of all means aimed at reducing the impact of disabling conditions and enabling the person with disabilities to achieve optimal social integration (Physical and Rehabilitation Medicine-WHO 1988). Mohandas Karamchand Gandhi (Bapu-Mahatma Gandhi), Father of the Nation (India), a freedom fighter, gave many life philosophies. One of them is "Self-sufficiency—Independence" (Fig. 1).

Rehabilitation professionals use this principle very well and make the disabled-dependent person "Self-sufficient" in communication,

Rehabilitation medicine means to make the disabled "independent" and "self sufficient" in all aspects of life

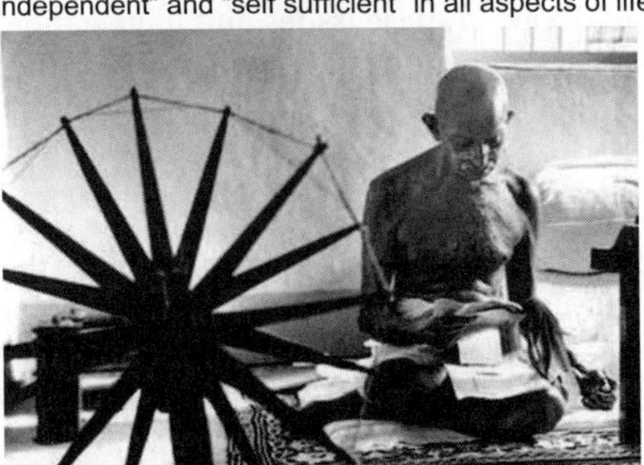

Fig. 1: Gandhian philosophy of vocational self-sufficiency

mobility, feeding, self-care, earning or learning for a life with liberty and pursuit of happiness).

Basic philosophy of rehabilitation is the "acceptance" of the disability by the person, set the goals and then efforts by patients, supported by Rehab professionals so as with a "Hope" to reach to a "Satisfying -Productive" post-injury "Independent and Self-sufficient" lifestyle.

Patient's thinking is harnessed and is motivated to achieve the Goal of "Independent, Interdependent and Integrated" human being in the family and the society.

A person with the impairment has the same basic rights and needs as any other person in the society. The rights, needs and cultural diversity of the family and support system are always considered. Patient's customized program is designed to maximize the individual's activities and participation in the environment, outside the hospital/ rehab setup. All efforts by the rehab team members are directed towards making the disabled person "Self-sufficient" and independent in the activities of daily living (ADL) with physical, mental, vocational, social and spiritual independence.

Need of Rehabilitation

The disabled person, due to disease or damage, loses his or her functions. After the recovery phase is over, the person is on rehabilitation process and with his available potentials, is made independent in the day-to-day activities. If not, some other person will have to take care for his personal and professional (earning) needs. The person becomes a burden to the family, society and the nation at large. To avoid these issues and to give independent and meaningful life, rehabilitation of disabled persons is needed and it is a right of the person.

Principles of Rehabilitation Medicine

The rehab process is unique in a sense that along with, medical and therapeutic measures many other aspects like psychology, sociology, vocational, educational and also patients, care taker, NGO are involved and integrated to take the disabled person to the desired destination of "Non-dependent" living.

Many "natural physical agents" are used in the treatment and management of rehab process: (1) Heat, (2) Cold, (3) Light, (4) Sun

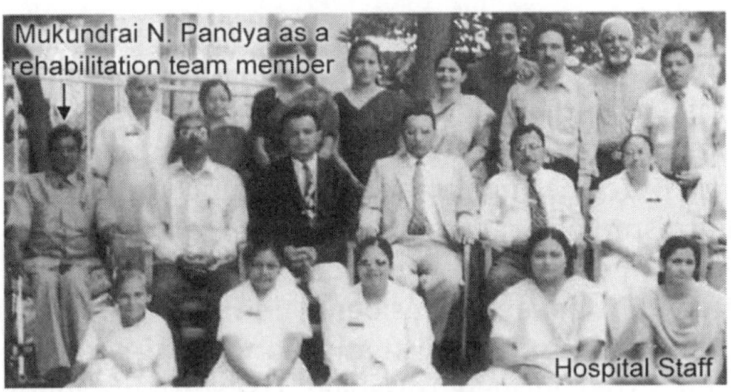

Fig. 2: Rehabilitation medicine team

rays, (5) Electricity, (6) Tailor-made designed therapeutic exercises, (7) Supportive and assistive Orthotic devices, (8) Human help, (9) Mind of a patient, (10) Team work in harmony.

Patient's thinking is harnessed and is motivated to achieve the goal of an independent human of the family and society. Patient is the active achiever of the goals and not the passive recipient of the rehab program.

Rehabilitation Medicine Team (Fig. 2)

Physical medicine and rehabilitation needs a well-coordinated team approach. The team members include: patient, care giver, family and friends, orthopedic surgeon, physical therapist, occupational therapist, speech pathologist and audiologist, orthotic and prosthetic engineer, rehab nurse, medical social worker, vocational counsellor, clinical psychologist, psychiatrist, neurologist, urologist, non-government organization (NGO).

IMPAIRMENT-DISABILITY-HANDICAP

International Classification of Disease (ICD) (Etiology > Pathology > Manifestations)

ICD provides a valuable and relevant means for studying the health experience and underlying cause concept is additionally helpful.

International Classification of Impairment, Disability, Handicap (ICIDH-1980 by WHO) Disease/Damage > Impairment > Disability > Handicap.

IMPAIRMENT (I code) any loss or abnormality of physiological, psychological, anatomical structures or functions, e.g. loss of a finger, loss of conduction of an impulse, loss of certain chemicals in brain leading to parkinsonism. Not all impairment lead to disability, e.g. loss of pinna of an ear would not lead to hearing loss but merely loss in cosmetic appearance. Impairment need not become handicap. Person can overcome impairment and can function fully (Impairment represents disturbance at organ level).

DISABILITY (D code) any restriction or loss of ability to perform an activity within the range considered normal for a person, resulting from an impairment, e.g. difficulty in walking after lower limb amputation. To be considered disabled, a person is not able to perform day to day activities normal for his age, sex and physique (Disability represent disturbance at the person level).

HANDICAP (H code) a disadvantage for a given individual in his/her social context, resulting from impairment or disability that limits or prevents from fulfillment of a role that is normal for that individual of his age, sex and physique. Many Socioeconomic factors like family background, financial status, living-learning earning, architectural set up, play a role in determining the handicap (Handicaps represent interactions-adaptations at social and surrounding level).

5

Rehabilitation Medicine Science Dimensions

- Institution-based Rehabilitation (IBR)
- Outreach-based Rehabilitation (OBR)
- Community-based Rehabilitation (CBR)
- Community approach to handicap in development (CAHD).

Institution-based Rehabilitation

Institution-based rehab (IBR) is a Rehab setup with a hospital (and a medical college at some places) or only outpatient clinic. The program is ideal and scientific in nature. The setup may also be attached with academic programs for rehab professionals and research projects are also follows on for a better care and cure for future. The focus of the control is based in the institute. This service meets needs of a small number of disabled persons. This is at best a limited approach and at worst it can abuse the rights of many other deprived disabled.

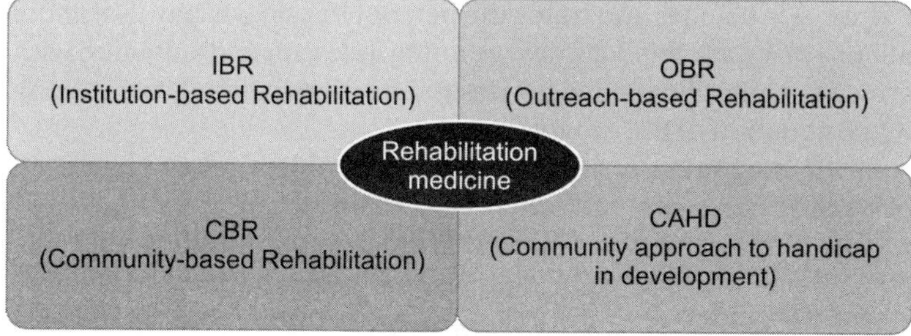

Fig. 1: Rehabilitation medicine

Outreach-based Rehabilitation

Outreach-based rehab (OBR)—the institutional-based rehab professional "reach out" to the disabled in their community in the form of Medical camps or Door step visits to patient's home for disabled screening, assessment, guidance and primary care. The focus of the control is still based in the Institution. More people can be "reached" but there will be limits according to the distance from the Institution, schedules, and according to whether the needs of disabled people is similar to what Institution offers.

Community-based Rehabilitation

Community-based rehab (CBR) is to help people with disabilities, by establishing community-based programs for social integration, equalization of opportunities. The professional rehab services are available in the urban areas and the rural disabled population is deprived of these services. This scenario is more or less in the developed and underdeveloped countries. The strength of the CBR is that they can be made available in rural areas with limited infrastructure (Utilization of the resources from within the community-persons and property). CBR programs involve the people with disability, their families, communities as well appropriate professionals. For example, mother of a cerebral palsy (CP) patient, SCI patient himself or his care taker. It involves preparation of simple gadgets/adaptations utilizing the material from that area, e.g. preparing a crutch from bamboo. The rehab professionals find out the appropriate patient or person from the family or a relevant professional from the community. Rehab professional develops tailored made, simple but scientific rehab program. He teaches and trains the person. Physio will pay visit at the patient's place at a regular interval, doing assessment/evaluation with corrections, modification in the designed program, finally convincing for continuation of the program.

In the beginning of 1960s, efforts to establish rehab centers in developing countries had taken hold of, in urban areas but failed to assist disabled persons in rural areas throughout the world. The first CBR pilot projects were launched in 1970s, and their continuing success led to CBR programs being adopted throughout Africa, Asia and South America.

Community Approach to Handicap in Development

Community approach to handicap in development (CAHD) is a program concept that was developed in Bangladesh by the Center for Disability in Development (CDD) in collaboration with Handicap International (HI).

Community—a group of people who lead and lives a life with certain beliefs and so their attitudes, e.g. in India in the past era, in certain province, people believed that alive wife should sit with her dead husband's body on cremation. This belief and attitude with an act was removed by the then social activist, Raja Ram Mohan Rai. Similar beliefs also exist in the community that the disability is a punishment given by God and the disabled person need not be treated. People in the community have a low level image about the disabled. Their potentials for performance are also thought to be poor. Instead of "Sympathy" they need "Empathy", "Encouragement" and "Empowerment". Instead of "disabled" these "differently-abled" needs "legal rights" as well, for the Rehab process and also for their rest of the life. There is also discriminative attitude towards the disabled in the society in many parts of the world. All these attitude needs to be altered and these differently able should have equal rights for their life and living. There are legal laws (Atrocity law) for calling-scolding a disabled.

Development work is primarily focused on eradication of poverty and on changing the attitudes and practices of the community. CAHD recognizes the impairment and disability as integral to development issues due to their close connection to poverty and aims to include them in the ongoing activities of mainstream development organization.

How CAHD Works

- **Knowledge:** Changing perspective requires creation of knowledge by providing information and creating experience. In CAHD, this information transfer is called social communication and experience gained through participating in inclusive activities. Also awareness can be achieved through media
- **Attitude:** Once knowledge is assimilated and combined with experience, it results in specific attitudes or ways of thinking about certain topics

- **Practice:** Ultimately, this newly-found knowledge and way of thinking will change practice. This is the key objective of CAHD.

DIFFERENCES BETWEEN THE IBR AND CBR

No.	*Aspect*	*IBR*	*CBR*
1	Location	Cities and Institutions	Anywhere in the community
2	Program	Rigid or a blue print	Flexible as per resources
3	Focus	Mainly on physical and medical needs	Active involvement of family and community as well
4	Care	Short-term residential	Partnership with disabled persons
5	Service	Delivering to disabled as passive recipient	Capacity building of disabled person and their family in the context of their community and culture
6	Approach	Physical, Mental	Holistic- multisectoral- social, employment, educational as well
7	Services	In isolation	In their own
8	Cost of care	Very costly	community Low cost
9	Machines	High-tech	Simple machines and gadgets
10	Decisions	Service provider	Disabled and their family as well
11	Service provider	Highly qualified many professionals	Disabled, family, CBR worker, semi-professional
12	Action	Usually responsive	Proactive
13	Complications	Easy to ease	Difficult to deal
14		Services plus scientific search for better care, (today and tomorrow)	Serving with present resources from the society (today)
15		Advancement of profession	Utilization of available resources

Institution-based rehab is useful for the growth of the profession with education of the "future" professionals and research whereas CBR is needed to provide service to the disabled with "present" available resources.

2

Section

Investigations
(Causes, Signs and Symptoms, Classifications and Investigations)

Chapter Outline

"SPINAL CORD INJURY (SCI) refers to any injury to the spinal cord that is caused by trauma instead of disease (Taber's Medical Dictionary). Depending on where the spinal cord and nerve roots are diseased or damaged with destructions, the symptoms can vary widely, from pain to paralysis. SCI is described at various levels of "Incomplete" which can vary from having minor or no effects on patients to "Complete" injury means total loss of function below the injury. Loss of functioning (sensory/motor) of anal sphincter S4–S5 indicates "complete lesion."

6

Causes of Spinal Cord Injury

TRAUMATIC

The trauma causes fracture of vertebrae and/or dislocation leading to the injury to the cord or occlusion of blood vessels. SCI is associated with trauma.

- Road traffic accidents
- Falls, e.g. fall from a tree, a pole, a house
- Work-related accidents
- Recreational sports, e.g. falling from horse, water or ski diving injury
- Violence, stabs, gunshot injury
- Sports injuries
- Whiplash injury.

The trauma causes lateral bending, rotation, axial loading, hyperflexion followed by hyperextension (e.g. whiplash injury— carrying heavy weight on head and there is sudden halt or a car moving with high speed and a sudden brake causes jerk to the body, moving the head forward and backwards like a whip. The neurological symptoms are observed without bony injury on X-ray) (Fig. 1).

The cord is injured by transection, distraction, compression, ischemia and bruises. Concussion can lead to temporary loss of function for hours or weeks. Some areas are inherently more vulnerable than others because of their relatively high mobility and less stability, e.g. C5–C6 in cervical and T12–L1 in thoracolumbar region. Thoracic spine with ribcage is more stable. More than 80% men are with SCI, usually men under 30 years of age.

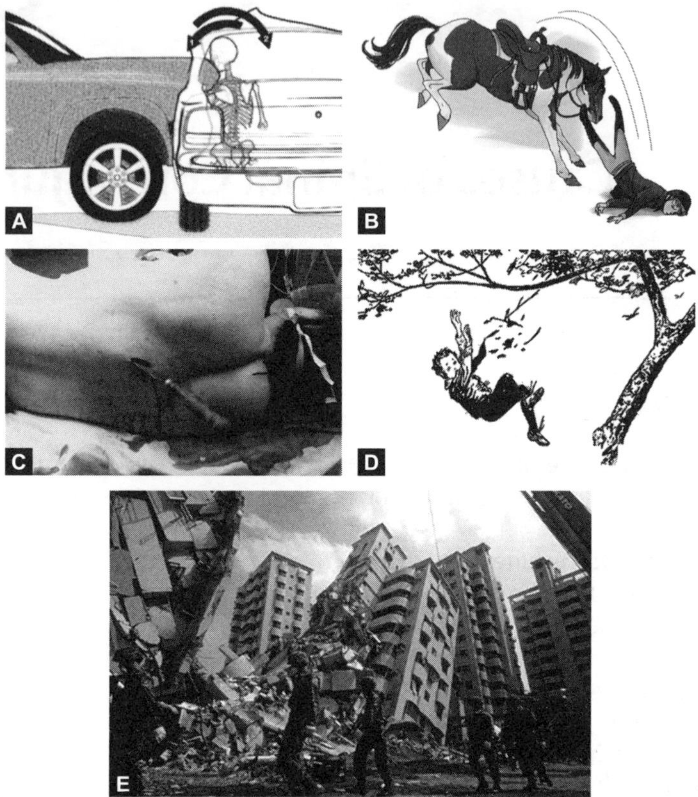

Figs 1A to E: Traumatic: (A) Road traffic accident simulation showing injury to the neck; (B) Falling on the neck from the horse; (C) Knife stab injury in the back may cause spinal cord injury; (D) Fall from a tree/roof/height may lead to spinal cord injury; (E) Massive damage caused by earthquake leading to multiple injuries to a lot of people (including spinal cord injury)

Pathophysiology

Primary injury occurs at the time of the traumatic insult. Secondary injury is due to poor handling of patient, delayed interventions inflammatory process, intracellular calcium changes leading to edema or ischemia.

NONTRAUMATIC

- Tumors, such as meningioma, astrocytoma, metastatic cancer
- Ischemia from occlusion of blood vessels, e.g. aneurysm, emboli, arteriosclerosis
- Developmental disorders, such as spina bifida
- Neurodegenerative diseases—Friedreich's ataxia, spinocerebellar ataxia
- Demyelinative diseases—Multiple sclerosis
- Inflammations—Transverse myelitis, tuberculosis, poliomyelitis
- Vascular malformations—Arteriovenous malformation, arterio-venous fistula
- Stenosis fluorosis.

7

Signs and Symptoms of Spinal Cord Injury

"Signs" are recorded by medical professionals and "symptoms" are experienced and narrated by patients, vary according to the level and extent of spinal cord injury.

Pain, numbness and loss of sensation in certain area suggest the "dermatomes" level whereas uncontrolled muscle contractions, weakness or complete paralysis in specific area suggest "myotome" level.

- Topographic classification (level of lesion): Higher the level, more paralysis to the body parts. In cervical lesions, all four limbs are involved (quadriplegia). Whereas in lower lesions in thoracic and lumbar, lower limbs are involved (paraplegia)
- Physiological classification "spastic" paralysis in upper motor neuron lesion (UMNL) and "flaccid" paralysis in lower motor neuron paralysis (LMNP)
- Severity of injury: Partial injury has some of the tracts of spinal cord intact, hence they continue their work of passing the messages to and from the body parts and brain. Complete lesions show complete loss of motor and sensory functioning.

SPINAL SHOCK

Definition

Temporary areflexia with loss of automatic control that may last up to 3–6 weeks postinjury is considered as spinal shock. Return of reflexes "bulbocavernosus" is typically the first to return and is the sign of resolution of shock and recovery. Functional recovery may take place as per the injury once the shock is over with the therapeutic measures.

Spinal shock was first described by Wyatt in 1750 as a loss of sensation accompanied by motor paralysis with initial loss of but gradual return of reflexes with sensation and motor power following SCI. The reflexes above the lesion are unaffected whereas below the lesion are absent (areflexia) or depressed (hyporeflexia). The shock starts within a few minutes and lasts up to 3–6 weeks (may last longer). Often person's loss of movement and sensation below the lesion may appear complete soon after the injury. This may mask real extent of damage. After few weeks, some of body's systems get adjusted and their function improves.

The mechanism of spinal shock involves the sudden loss of conduction in the spinal cord as a result of migration of potassium from the intracellular to extracellular spaces. This is associated with the transient loss of somatic and autonomic reflexes below the lesion. The spinal cord reflex arc immediately above the lesion may also be disrupted. The return of reflexes indicates the recovery from the spinal shock, the "bulbocavernosus" reflex typically first to return. Some clinicians classify the end of shock with return of deep reflexes or reflexive detrusor function, which may be months after the injury.

Bulbocavernosus (BCR) or bulbospongiosus reflex is tested by mechanical stimulation of glans penis or vulva or tugging of Foley's catheter and monitoring anal sphincter contractions. The reflex involves the S2–4 nerve root and is a spinal cord mediated reflex arc. Absence of BCR with sensory loss in perineal area indicates complete injury.

In cases of cervical or thoracic cord injury, absence of BCR reflex documents continuation of spinal shock or spinal cord injury at the reflex arc itself. Spinal shock does not apply to the lesions that occurs below the cord and, therefore, the low lumbar burst fracture, should not cause spinal shock and in this situation the absence of the BCR indicates that there is a cauda equina injury. Persistent loss of the BCR is a result of conus medullaris injury.

NEUROGENIC SHOCK

Definition

A circulatory disease with hypotension as a result of bradycardia and vasodilatation due to loss of thoracic sympathetic innervation following cord injury is considered neurogenic shock.

It can result from severe CNS damage, brain, cervical or high thoracic injury. The trauma causes a sudden loss of background sympathetic stimulation to the blood vessels. This will cause vasodilation, resulting in sudden decrease in blood pressure (hypotension), secondary to peripheral vascular resistance and pooling of blood in the extremities. Bradycardia (slow heart rate) occurs due to unopposed vagal activity with hypoxia (oxygen deficiency) and endobronchial suction. The limbs are warm and rest of the body is cold (hypothermia), cardiac output (the amount of blood that heart pumps out at every contraction) is reduced. Neurogenic shock is a life-threatening situation and needs immediate medical emergency attention otherwise it can lead to dysfunction or death.

Neurological shock is different from spinal shock in a way that spinal shock is not circulatory in nature.

8

Classifications of Spinal Cord Injury

There are many classifications for spinal cord injury. They are as follows:

- Frankel
- ASIA (widely used)
- Nurick
- Ranawat
- Chiles
- Japanese Orthopaedic Association (JOA)

FRANKEL'S SCALE (FIG. 1)

Frankel's scale was introduced in 1971.

- Grade A: Complete neurological injury—No motor or sensory function
- Grade B: Preserved partial sensation (sacral sparing only), no motor function
- Grade C: Preserved nonfunctional motor function (no practical use)
- Grade D: Preserved useful motor function. Patient can walk with deviated gait
- Grade E: Normal motor-sensory and sphincter function. Abnormal reflexes.

ASIA SCALE

American Spinal Injury Association (ASIA) scale was introduced in 1982. The American Spinal Injury Association published its first International classification in 1982, a modified Frankel's scale and is

A = **Complete.** No sensory or motor function is preserved in the sacral segments S4–S5.
B = **Incomplete.** Sensory but not motor function is preserved below the neurological level and includes the sacral segments S4–S5.
C = **Incomplete.** Motor function is preserved below the neurological level, and more than half of key muscles below the neurological level have a muscle grade less than 3.
D = **Incomplete.** Motor function is preserved below the neurological level, and at least half of key muscles below the neurological level have a muscle grade greater than or equal to 3.
E = **Normal.** Sensory and motor function is normal.

Fig. 1: Frankel's scale

widely used to document sensory and motor impairment following SCI. It is based on neurological responses.

- Dermatomes—Touch and pin-prick sensation tested in each "Dermatomes"
  - 0 = Absent
  - 1 = Impaired
  - 2 = Normal
  - NT = Not testable.
- Myotomes—The strength of the muscles that control ten key motions. Muscle strength gradations (for lower motor lesions):
  - 0 = No contractions, total paralysis
  - 1 = Visible or palpable contractions
  - 2 = Active full range of motion, gravity eliminated
  - 3 = Active full range of motion against gravity
  - 4 = Active full range of motion against gravity with some resistance
  - 5 = Active full range of motion against gravity with full resistance (Normal)
  - NT = Not testable.
- Voluntary control at joint (Muscle charting is at muscle level, Voluntary control is at joint level)
  - Nil = No movement possible
  - Poor = Some initiation of movement
  - Fair = Movement in gravity eliminated plane
  - Good = Movement against gravity
  - Normal = Movement against gravity plus resistance.
- Spasticity gradation modified Ashworth scale (MAS) is simple and is reproducible. MAS measures resistance on passive soft tissue

stretching. MAS is graded with the "gravity speed "(same speed as nonspastic limb would naturally drop. Faster speed increases spasticity).

- 0 = No increase in muscle tone
- 1 = Slight increase in muscle tone with a catch or resistance at the end of range
- 1+ = A catch and minimal resistance throughout range (less than half)
- 2 = More marked increase in tone throughout range but part is easily moved
- 3 = Considerable increase in tone, passive movement difficult
- 4 = Affected part rigid in that position.

"Ten" muscle groups represent the motor innervation by cervical and lumbosacral spinal cord. The ASIA system does not include the abdominal muscles because the thoracic levels are easier to determine from sensory levels. It also excludes certain muscles (e.g. Hamstrings) because the segmental levels that innervate them are already represented by other muscles.

A	Arm and hand muscles
	C5: Elbow flexors (biceps)
	C6: Wrist extensors
	C7: Elbow extensors (triceps)
	T1: Little finger abductor
B	Leg and foot muscles
	L2: Hip flexors (psoas)
	L3: Knee extensors (quadriceps)
	L4: Ankle dorsi flexors(tibialis anterior)
	L5: Long toe extensors (extensor hallucis longus)
	S1: Ankle plantar flexors (gastrocnemius)
C	Anal sphincter is innervated by the S4–S5. It represents the end of the cord. The anal sphincter is a critical part of spinal cord injury examination. If the person has no sensory deficit and voluntary anal contraction, regardless of any other findings, that person is by definition a motor "incomplete" injury.

"ASIA" Impairment Scale

- A: Indicates a "complete" spinal cord injury where no motor or sensory function is preserved in the sacral segment S4–S5

- B: Indicates an "incomplete" spinal cord injury where sensation is present but not motor function below the neurological level and includes the sacral segments S4–S5. This is typically a transient phase and if the person recovers any motor function below the neurological level, that person essentially becomes a motor incomplete, i.e. ASIA C or D
- C: Indicates an "incomplete" spinal cord injury where motor function is preserved below the neurological level and more than half of key muscles have a muscle grade less than 3
- D: Indicates an "incomplete" spinal cord injury where motor function is preserved below the neurological level and more than half of the key muscles below the lesion have muscle grade 3 and more.
- E: Indicates "normal" where motor and sensory scores are normal. Note that it is possible to have spinal cord injury and neurological deficits with completely normal neurological scores.

Spinal cord injury of any kind may result in with one or more signs and symptoms.

- Pain—intense stinging sensation caused by the damaged nerve fibers in the cord
- Loss of motor movement
- Loss of sensation (pain, touch, proprioception, temperature) below the level
- Loss of sweating below the lesion
- Loss of sphincter control with bladder-bowel dysfunction
- Exaggerated reflex activity, spasticity
- Changes in sexual sensitivity and functioning
- Difficulty in breathing, coughing and clearing secretions from lungs
- Additional associated disorders (Patient may have additional problems, if other body parts are injured, e.g. unconsciousness with head injury).

NURICK SCALE

A six grade system (0–5) based on the 'difficulty in walking'.

Classification Scheme:

- Grade 0: signs or symptoms of root involvement but without evidence of spinal cord disease

- Grade 1: signs of spinal cord disease but no difficulty in walking.
- Grade 2: slight difficulty in walking which does not prevent full-time employment
- Grade 3: difficulty in walking which prevented full time employment or the ability to do all housework, but which was not so severe as to require someone else's help to walk
- Grade 4: able to walk only with someone else's help or with the aid of a frame.
- Grade 5: chairbound or bedridden.

Ranawat Classification of Neurologic Deficit

Classification

- Class I: Pain, no neurologic deficit
- Class II: Subjective weakness, hyperreflexia, dysesthesias
- Class III: Objective weakness, long tract signs
  - Class IIIA: Ambulatory
  - Class IIIB: Nonambulatory

Japanese Orthopaedic Association Classification

A point scoring system (17 total) based on function in the following categories:

- Upper extremity motor function
- Lower extremity motor function
- Sensory function
- Bladder function

9

Level of Lesion and Dysfunction

CERVICAL

- C1–C2—results in loss of breathing, needs mechanical ventilator or phrenic nerve pacing
- C3 and above—results in loss of breathing, needs mechanical ventilator
- C4—results in significant loss in functions of biceps and shoulder
- C5—results in potential loss in functions of biceps and shoulder and complete loss of function at wrist and hand
- C6—results in limited loss of wrist control; complete loss of functions of hand
- C7–T1—results in lack of dexterity in the hands and fingers, but allows for limited use of arm. Patients with complete lesions above C7 cannot handle ADL (activities of daily livings), independent functioning is difficult.

Additional signs and symptoms of cervical injury:

- Inability or reduced ability to regulate heart rate, blood pressure, sweating and body temperature
- Autonomic dysreflexia or abnormal increase in blood pressure, sweating and disturbance in other autonomic responses to pain and sensations.

THORACIC

Complete injury at or below the thoracic spinal level results in paraplegia, incomplete lesions ends in paraparesis. Functions of breathing, hands, arms and neck is not affected in general.

- T1–T8—Inability to control the abdominal muscles and hence trunk stability is affected. Lower the lesion, lesser the effect on trunk stability. T6 and above lesions causes typical autonomic dysreflexia
- T9–T12—Partial loss of trunk and abdominal muscles control.

LUMBOSACRAL

Lumbosacral lesion of spinal cord causes decreased control of legs, hips, bladder and bowel. Bladder and bowel function is regulated by the sacral region of the spine. Patient may experience dysfunction of bladder and bowel including bladder infection and bowel incontinence.

Designation of level of lesion—American Spinal Injury Association (ASIA) and International Standards of Neurological Classification of Spinal Cord Injury (ISNCSCI) have standardized to determine, define and document the level as the most caudal level of the spinal cord with normal motor and sensory function on both sides of body.

10

Sexuality in Spinal Cord Injury

Persons with spinal cord injury (SCI) are in general in their peak of youth around 30 years of age. Sexual thoughts and sexual activities are most important part of their day-to-day life. With the problems of penile erection, pelvic and whole body mobility, person with SCI finds it extremely difficult to perform sexual acts which are very distressing. Such persons need to be educated on issues like adjustments with disability, adaptations, alternative options for sexual act and sexual pleasure.

Adaptations to the disability by SCI takes a prolonged period of time, successful sexual adjustment is also one of the dimensions of adjustment. Sexual adjustments are influenced by the level and severity of lesion, physical health, age, gender, social support, care and comforts at home. For satisfying sexual gratifications, the SCI person should have proper knowledge and information about the disability—problems, sexual options, adaptations and adjustments. Many persons with SCI will remain focused on ambulation and regaining functions and will neglect about sexual issues. Even if the person does not initiate about this issue, the rehabilitation team members, must provide basic information about erection, ejaculation, orgasm, lubrication, positioning, sensation and cleanliness of the genital area and to remain well dressed and attractive.

Providing sexual education to individuals with SCI and their partners is best accomplished by an interdisciplinary team approach in which physical, medical and psychological issues can be addressed.

MALE SEXUALITY

Erectile and ejaculatory functions are complex involving psychological, and physiological activities that require interaction between the vascular, nervous and endocrine systems.

Erection is controlled by the parasympathetic nervous system (PNS). Somatic afferent fibers travel from cauda equina, exit from S2–S4 of spinal cord and through the Pudendal nerve, reach the genital region. The postganglion parasympathetic fibers secrete nitric oxide, which causes relaxation of the smooth muscles of the corpus cavernosum and increases blood flow to the penile arteries. Consequently, the vascular chambers of the penis become engorged with the blood, and the result is an erection. This reflex is modulated by brainstem, subcortical and cortical centers. In addition, the erectile function is influenced by the testosterone hormone.

Ejaculation is the climax stage of male sexual act and is controlled by the sympathetic nervous system. Similar to the sympathetic innervations of the bladder, these fibers originate in the thoraco-lumbar spinal cord and travel into the sympathetic chain. These impulses then travel through the splanchnic nerves into the hypogastric plexus. After synapsing into the inferior mesenteric ganglion, postganglionic fibers travel through the hypogastric nerve to supply the vas deferens, seminal vesicles and ejaculatory ducts in the prostate.

Sexual function is associated with sacral spinal segment and is generally affected in men with SCI.

Erectile capacity is greater in

- Upper motor lesions than lower motor lesions
- Incomplete lesions than complete lesions.

Ejaculation is higher in

- Lower motor than upper motor lesions
- Lower level versus upper level lesions
- Incomplete as compared to complete lesions.

Psychogenic erections—Sexual thoughts from the brain go down the descending tracts and signals reach to the sacral parasympathetic cell bodies at spinal level S2–S4, where they are relayed for erection of penis (So, in cases of lesions above S2–S4, psychogenic erection will not occur).

Reflexogenic erection—Patients with lesions above S2–S4, reflexogenic erections can be achieved by physical contacts/ stimulating genital organs (So, in cases of lesions at S2–S4, reflexogenic erection is also impaired).

Ejaculation—In men with SCI, the ability to ejaculate is less common than the ability of erection. The rate of ejaculation varies with the level and severity of the lesion. Many men who can ejaculate, experience the retrograde ejaculation in the bladder with dribbling of semen.

Orgasm—The experience of orgasm in men with SCI varies. Some narrate it as an emotional event, other it as a generalized relaxation around pelvic area and pleasant sensation. Some report it as nonexistent.

MALE FERTILITY

Majority of men with all levels of SCI experience difficulty to have child through the impregnation of an egg during sexual intercourse. This is due to erectile and ejaculation dysfunction and poor semen quality. Disability worries also affect the sexual desire which may also affect the arousal, sexual performance and frequency of sexual intercourse.

With ejaculatory difficulty, men with SCI must often use techniques rather than intercourse to achieve impregnation of female's egg. These are manual stimulation, use of penile vibratory stimulation or an electrorectal probe to get semen sample.

After obtaining the semen sample and determining the quality of semen, the couple can go for fertility with various methods including: (1) Intravaginal insemination, (2) Intrauterine insemination, (3) In vitro fertilization, (4) Gamete intrafallopian transfer.

Men with SCI have fragile sperm that lose their ability to swim. Although they have normal number of sperms, SCI have 20% of motile sperms compared to men without injury.

URINARY AND FECAL INCONTINENCE

Bladder and bowel accidents may occur at any time during courtship, sexual activity, at workplace and in social events which is a major fear for social rejection and sexual act in the minds of persons with SCI.

To minimize the untimely episodes of incontinence, the bladder and bowel (removal with a finger) should be emptied prior to the sexual act. Foley's catheter can be taped to the side of penis with a condom on the catheter, and in case of female, catheter to be taped on abdomen. Gentle thrusting, coital positioning and a careful food and fluid intake to reduce accidents. Towel should be available in cases of incontinence. Couple needs to discuss these issues of their feelings and fear.

FEMALE SEXUALITY

Female sexual satisfaction is with the interactions of endocrine and nervous system. Psychogenic and physical stimulation provide sexual excitement. The arousal is manifested by vaginal lubrication and tightening of introitus. Stimulation of genital region including the clitoris, labia majora and labia minora causes afferent signals to travel via pudendal nerve in to S2–S4 segments of the spinal cord. These fibers interact with the efferent parasympathetic fibers that project through the pelvic nerve. There is dilatation of perineal muscles and tightening of introitus. Parasympathetic fibers cause the Bartholin's gland to secrete mucus for vaginal lubrication.

Female orgasm is characterized by rhythmic contractions of pelvic structures. Female orgasm also results in cervical dilatation which may aid in sperm transportation and fertility. Most women with SCI can achieve some level of vaginal lubrication similar to penile erection in male. It is mediated by reflexogenic or psychogenic factors.

- *Psychological erection of clitoris*—Sexual thoughts from the brain go down the descending tracts and signals reach to the sacral parasympathetic cell bodies at the spinal level S2–S4,where they are relayed for erection of clitoris (so in cases of lesions above S2–S4, psychogenic erection will not occur)
- *Reflexogenic erection of clitoris*—Patients with lesions above S2–S4, reflexogenic erections can be achieved by physical contacts/stimulating genital organs (so in cases of lesions at S2–S4, reflexogenic erection is also impaired).

Women with incomplete lesion (both upper and lower motor neuron) are more likely to get satisfactory lubrication. If vaginal lubrication is unsatisfactory, water-soluble lubrication is recommended.

FEMALE FERTILITY

Menstruation usually returns within 6 months postinjury. Neither the level nor the completeness of lesion affects menstruation. Most women are fertile with SCI and the couple should use birth control techniques unless they desire a child.

BIRTH CONTROL

Condoms provide the birth control as well as diminish the risk of sexually transmitted diseases (STD). Oral contraception containing only progesterone is safer. The intrauterine device (IUD) may be associated with increased incidences of pelvic inflammatory diseases (PID) and autonomic dysreflexia. Women with SCI may not be able to perceive if the device has migrated from the cervix.

PREGNANCY

Spinal cord injury pregnant women have risk of urinary tract infection (UTI), leg edema, autonomic dysreflexia, constipation, thromboembolism and premature birth. Since uterine innervation arises from T10– T12, patients with T10 and above lesions may not perceive uterine contraction or fetal movements. It may be difficult to differentiate between pregnancy-induced hypertension (preeclampsia) and autonomic dysreflexia. During second and third trimester pregnant woman may find difficulty in performing functional task independently that was possible previously. Transfers may require assistance of care giver and powered wheel chair (WC) for mobility.

11

Clinical Syndromes

Some incomplete lesions have distinct clinical pictures with signs and symptoms. An understanding of the various syndromes can be helpful to the client's team in planning the Rehabilitation program.

CENTRAL CORD SYNDROME

"Hyperextension" injury usually results in a central cord syndrome (Fig. 1). It also has been associated with the congenital or degenerating narrowing of the spine. The resultant compressive forces give rise to hemorrhage or edema, producing damage to the most central aspect of the cord. This injury causes bleeding into the central gray matter resulting in more impairment of the functions of upper extremities than the lower extremities. Varying degrees of sensory impairment occur but tend to be less severe than the motor deficit. These patients are generally known as "walking quadru".

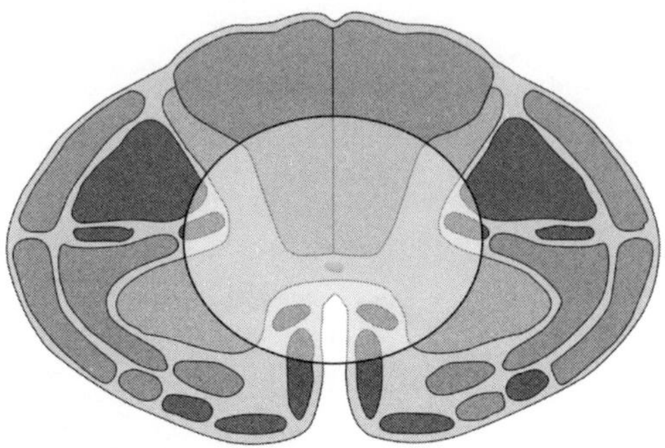

Fig. 1: Central cord syndrome

ANTERIOR CORD SYNDROME

Anterior cord syndrome (Fig. 2) is frequently related to "flexion" injuries of cervical region with resultant damage to the anterior portion of the cord and/or its vascular supply from anterior spinal artery. This syndrome is characterized by loss of motor function and loss of sense of pain and temperature below the level of the lesion. Proprioception, kinesthesia and vibratory sense are generally preserved.

BROWN SEQUARD SYNDROME

Brown sequard syndrome (Fig. 3) occurs from the "hemisection" of the spinal cord (Damage to right or left side of the cord). It is typically caused by stab wound injury. Partial lesion occurs more frequently, true hemisections are rare. The clinical features are asymmetrical. On the ipsilateral (same) side of the lesion, there is loss of sensation in the

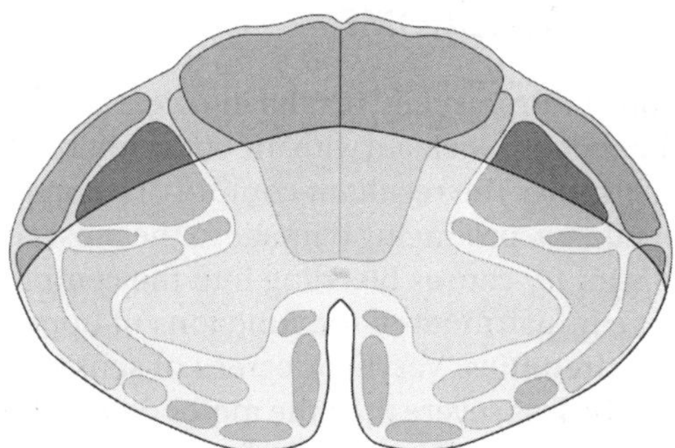

Fig. 2: Anterior cord syndrome

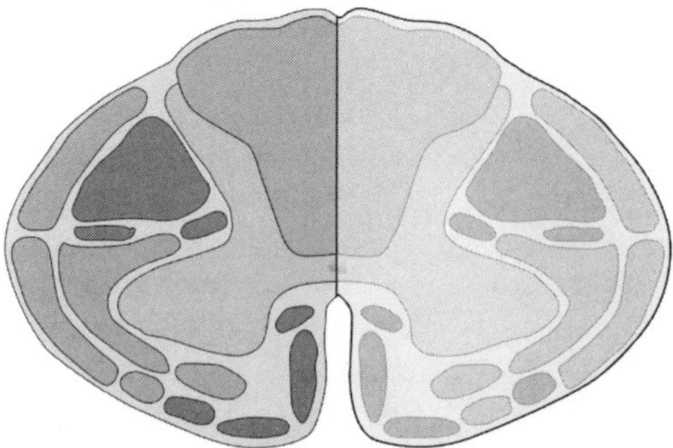

Fig. 3: Brown sequard syndrome

dermatome segment corresponding to the level of lesion. Owing to the lateral column damage, there are decreased reflexes, clonus, positive Babinski's sign. As a result of dorsal column damage, there is loss of proprioception, kinesthesia and vibratory sense. On the contralateral (opposite) side to the lesion, damage to the spinothalamic tract, results in loss of pain and temperature. The loss begins several dermatomes segments below the lesion. This discrepancy in level occurs because the lateral spinothalamic tract ascends 2–4 segments before crossing.

POSTERIOR CORD SYNDROME

Posterior cord syndrome (Fig. 4) is very rare, resulting from compression by tumor or infarction of the posterior spinal artery. Clinically proprioception, stereognosis, two point discrimination and vibratory sense are lost below the level of lesion. A wide base step gait pattern is typical.

CAUDA EQUINA SYNDROME

Damage to the cauda equina occurs with the injuries at the L1 vertebral level and below, resulting in a lower motor lesion, which is usually an incomplete lesion. This lesion results in flaccid paralysis. No spinal reflex activity is present.

SACRAL SPARING

Sacral sparing refers to an incomplete lesion in which the most centrally situated sacral tracts are spared. Varying levels of innervations from

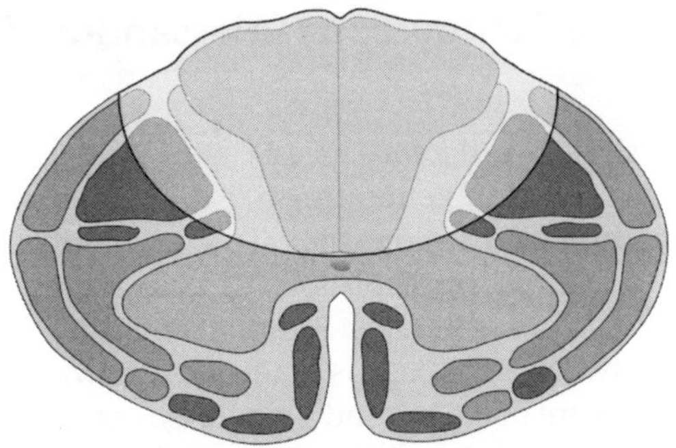

Fig. 4: Posterior cord syndrome

sacral segments remain intact. Clinical signs include present perineal sensation and external anal sphincter contraction.

CONUS MEDULLARIS SYNDROME

Injury to the sacral cord or lumbar nerve roots within neural canal, a clinical picture of lower extremity motor and sensory loss and areflexic bladder and bowel.

INVESTIGATIONS

Along with the clinical findings, following investigations are useful to establish the diagnosis, level of lesion with severity and the status of the systems functioning.

X-rays

X-rays is a form of radiation, like light or radiowaves that are focused into a beam, much like a flashlight beam (German physicist Roentgen in 1895). It has 0.01–10 nanometers as wavelength and frequency of 30 petahertz (3×10^{16}).

Dense tissues in the body, such as bones absorb many of X-rays and look white on X-ray film. Less dense tissues, such as muscles organs, block fewer of the X-rays (more X-rays pass through) and look shades of gray on an X-ray film. X-rays that pass only through air and look black on the film. X-ray shows damage or disease that affect the disks or joints in the spine, fractures of the bones, infections, tumors, dislocations, bone spurs, disk diseases and degenerations.

Computed Axial Tomography (Alessandro of Italy 1900s)

Tomography—Greek word *tomos* means "slice" and *graphein* means to write. It is a process of generating a 2-dimensional image on a slice or section through a 3-dimensional object; similar to looking at one slice of bread within the whole loaf. CT scan scanner uses digital geometry processing to generate a 3-dimensional (3D) image of the inside of the body. The 3D image is made after many 2-dimensional (2D) X-ray images are taken around a single axis of rotation. In other words, many pictures of the same area are taken from many angles and then placed together on computer to produce a 3D image.

A CT scan emits a series of narrow beams through human body as it moves through an arc, unlike an X-ray machine which sends just one radiation. The final picture is far more detailed than X-ray picture. Sometimes a contrast dye is used because it shows up much more clearly on the screen. A metal interferes with the working of the CT scan; the patient will need to remove all jewellery and metal fastening outside and inside the body.

Magnetic Resonance Imaging (Herman in 1952)

Magnetic resonance imaging (MRI) uses a magnetic field and pulses of radiowave energy to make pictures of organs and structures inside the body. In many cases, MRI gives different information about structures than can be seen with an X-ray, ultrasound, CT scan. MRI scan are digital images that can be saved and stored on a computer for a detailed study. The images also can be viewed remotely, such as in a clinic or an operating room. In some cases, contrast material may be used during the MRI scan to show certain structures more clearly. It shows location of lesion, status of soft tissues, reveals the problems of hematoma or blood clot (metal in/on body is unsafe)

Difference between MRI and CT scan

- A CT scan uses X-rays, MRI uses magnets and radiowaves
- A CT scan does not show tendons and ligaments, MRI does
- A CT scan shows organ tear and injury more quickly, so better in accident injury
- Broken bones and vertebrae are better seen on CT scan, soft tissues on MRI.

Ultrasonography (Dr George Ludwig Maryland US and John Wild in Late 1940s)

Ultrasonography is a noninvasive imaging technique that relies on detection of the reflections or echoes generated as high-frequency sound waves are passed into the body. It is used for investigations of abdominal and pelvic masses, cardiac echocardiography and prenatal fetal imaging. Less commonly, it has also been applied to detection of spinal and paraspinal disorders.

It can be used for degenerative disk diseases to determine whether back pain is a consequence of fissuring or herniation of the gelatinous disks that separate the vertebra. It is used also for injuries to paraspinal ligaments after spinal fractures.

Myelography

Contrast (dye that shows up on X-ray) is injected into the fluid-filled spaces between the bones. Dye is able to move through the space in order to allow the spinal cord and the nerve roots to see more clearly on X-ray. Myelography followed by CT scan is an alternative for patients who can not have an MRI scan, because they have a pacemaker or other implanted metallic device (rarely used).

Somatosensory-evoked Potential (SSEP)

This test evokes responses from nervous system upon stimulation. It can show if the nerve signals are able to pass through the spinal cord or if an injury is blocking the transmission.

EMG Study

Electromyography (EMG) is the study of electrical activities taking place in a muscle by needle on surface electrode of EMG machine at rest and during activities to find out the type of lesion and amount of innervations.

MRI/X-ray/CAT scan is the study of static structures whereas EMG is the dynamic study of electrical activities. However, nowadays functional MRI is being done.

NCV Study

It is a study of the speed of an impulse (thought wave) passing hrough the nerve. Both sensory and motor speed can be measured. The average speed is 45–75 meters/second. The speed is reduced in neuropathy, entrapment syndromes.

Laboratory Tests

As per need laboratory tests are carried out, namely—

- Blood-group, counts, hemoglobin, sugar, urea, cholesterol, erythrocyte sedimentation rate (ESR)
- Urine routine and culture
- Stool examination.

3 Section

Implementations (Management)

Chapter Outline

12

Prevention Plans

OCCUPATIONAL HAZARDS

If proper care is taken during the work, falls and many hazards can be prevented, thereby spinal cord injury (SCI) can also be prevented.

Traffic rules observance, if observed well, road traffic accident (RTA) can be prevented and thereby SCI can be prevented.

At the site—If proper care is taken, the injury severity can be minimized.

During transportation, if proper and prompt steps are taken, the intensity of the injury can be restricted with lesser problems and spinal brace.

Combinations of objective (science) with subjective (spiritual) forces are helpful. SCI need constant psychological support, sympathy and empathy of fellow feeling with medical and rehab services. All

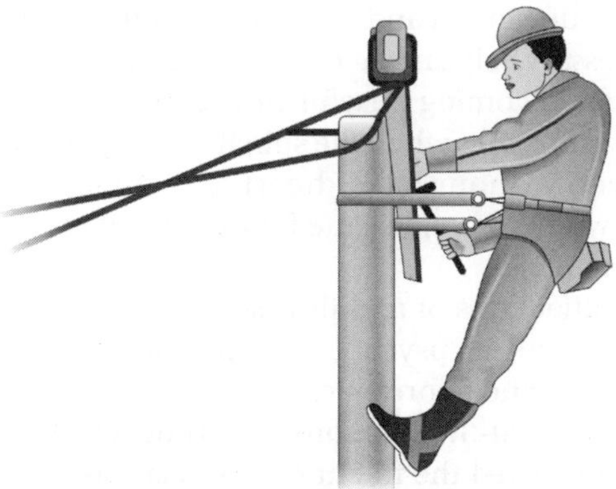

Fig. 1: Use of a safety belt to prevent falls

humans have "emotions". Patients and relatives are with "disturbed emotions." Patients are not machines and they need to be handled with following forces to provide positivity to patients' psychology, for better results without any set back or stagnancy.

- Force of love-affections and warmth for better relationship and rapport
- Force of faith, a firm foundation of the rehab program. Faith is the force of life
- Force of prayer reduces worries and improves efforts
- Force of touch provides assurance to the patient
- Force of kind words soothes patient and motivates patient. From the management point of view, these are two distinct stages but they overlap each other when needed.
- Survival team appears in the early phase
- Settlement team appears in the later phase, after the medical settlement.

There are five phases of management.

- Prehospital care
- Emergency room care
- Hospital and operative care
- Rehabilitative care
- Lifelong follow-up care.

The treatment of SCI starts at the site of an injury, site to service center and in the hospital, restraining the spine by orthosis and surgery to control the further damage and inflammation. The program continues with substantial physiotherapy, occupational therapy and rehabilitation for mobility and activities of daily living. Also psychosocial adjustment and vocational resettlement is taken care of. Lifelong necessary help and guidance is given to be with the family and community for becoming a useful independent citizen, on discharge.

"Frog instantly dies when the spinal cord is pierced, and previous to this it lived without head, heart, intestine, and bowel. Here, therefore, it would seem, lies the foundation of movement and life." Leonardo da Vinci.

With the affections of mobility, sensation, bladder, bowel along with economic, social, psychological perspective, the impact of SCI is encompassing and enormous.

Hippocrates (460–377 BC) considered both Father of medicine and orthopedic discussed the fractures/dislocations of spinal vertebrae and their correlation to SCI with chronic paralysis, constipation, bladder problem, bedsores. He believed that there is no reasonable therapy for SCI and they are "destined to die". He is credited with developing methods of reducing spinal deformities by administering traction with his extension bench, the "Scamnum". This device, with various modifications, has been used in the spinal disorder throughout the history and in present days. He hypothesized that cure may be feasible if anterior reduction of fracture is possible, a precursor to anterior surgical decompression.

Edwin Smith papyrus did the open reduction of spinal dislocation. Galen (131–201 AD) who followed the Hippocratic methods wrote on experimental physiology and mentioned about Brown-Sequard syndrome with hemisection.

The 18th century was characterized by surgeries. James (1745) advocated operative interventions for spinal dislocations. During 19th century, debate raged about the efficacy of surgery in SCI. Dr Albah Smith (1829) of US, successfully performed the lumbar laminectomy on a 2-year-old case of a person who fell from a horse with progressive paralysis. Postoperatively patient showed some recovery.

In the early era of 20th century, prognosis remained poor but it improved because of advances in bacteriology and disinfections by Pasteur and Lister and discovery of X-ray by Roentgen. Along with improved medical care, rehab measures with inclusion of socio, psycho, vocational aspects, SCI person's morbidity and mortality reduced. Many SCI patients can now enjoy a self-sufficient, satisfying meaningful life.

SCI patients were neglected in the past." An ailment not to be treated" and they are "destined to die" was the writing in medical literature. After the end of World War I, in early 1930, pioneering work was done by Dr Donald Munro of Boston, USA, developing specialized units for the treatment and rehabilitation of SCI. Dr Munro is the father of modern SCI care. Sir Ludwig "Poppa" Guttman (3rd July 1899–18th March 1980), a Jewish German born neurologist settled in Britain, established a unit at Stoke Mandeville UK on 1st February 1944 and introduced multidisciplinary staffing for the comprehensive treatment and rehab. This unit became world-renowned center for clinical care, teaching and research. Prof Guttman (Fig. 2) organized the first Stoke Mandeville games for disabled on 28th July 1948, the same day as the start of London 1948 summer Olympics. Later, it became "Paralympic" (Fig. 3).

In the present era, many new diagnostic techniques are developed, such as positive contrast myelography, radionuclide myelography, peridurography, angiography, discography, computerized axial tomography (CAT), magnetic resonance imaging (MRI), digital subtraction angiography, ultrasonography, EMG/NCV-electrophysiological studies, evoked potential (motor and sensory) and myelonoscopy.

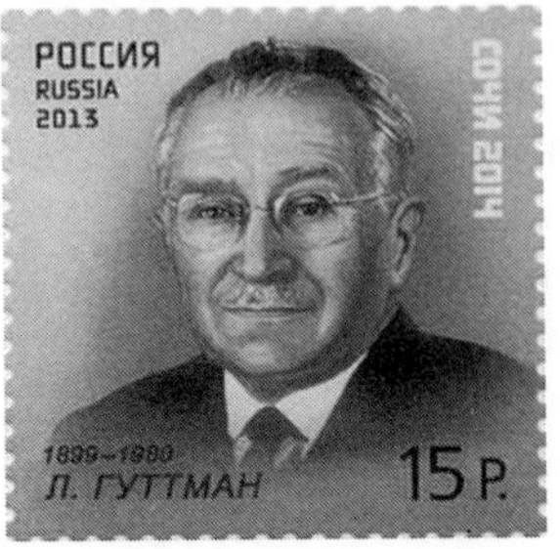

Fig. 2: Ludwig Guttmann on a 2013 Russian stamp from the series "Sports Legends" (*Source:* Wikipedia)

Advancement in medical, surgical and rehabilitation, has helped a lot to these victims.

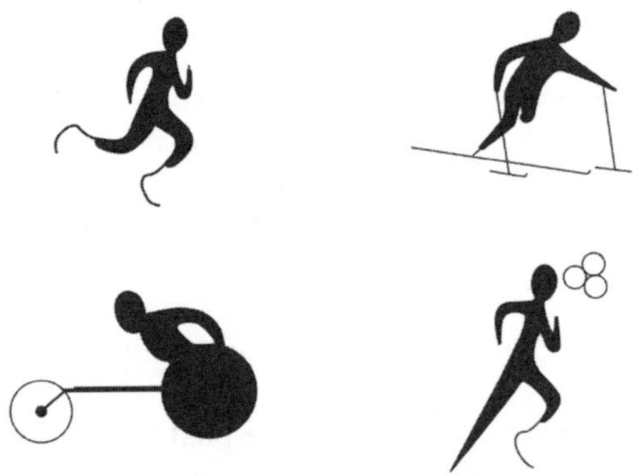

Fig. 3: Paralympic sports symbols

13

Prehospital Care

AT THE SITE AND DURING TRANSPORTATION

If you are at the accident scene: Treat the person as if that person has also suffered spinal cord injury until otherwise proven.

The first person to render aid or emergency care, if fail to take basic proper precautions, a minor or treatable condition can become permanent paralysis.

Following are some precautionary points to avoid further damage:

- Do not move victim unless they are in imminent danger, fire, leaking gas, etc.
- Support or brace the neck and back while moving. If the neck collar or back brace are not available than wrap and pin up a fourfold towel/coat/shirt around neck and fasten pillows in front and back of the spine
- Carefully lie a person down rather than in sitting position
- Do not turn or tilt the neck and back unless necessary for CPR. If turning is a must, the neck and back be moved like a log of wood
- Do not try to remove person's jacket or clothing
- Call emergency medical vehicle. Do not allow person to get up. Victims may lose functions or feelings, gradually or suddenly from swelling, leaking spinal fluids or suffer further damage due to movement.

TRANSPORTATION FROM SITE TO SERVICE CENTER

Prior to the extrication and transportation, from the site of accident to the hospital, person's medical condition is made stable with CPR or oxygen tube. The spine of a person needs to be immobilized in a natural vertebral alignment. The limbs with sensory loss need to be taken care from sharp and hot objects. They should be brought to hospital by trained emergency medical technicians (EMT) (Fig. 1). Person is placed on an "Extrication board" (a hard rescue board) with a cervical collar and spinal brace and transported (Fig. 2). If possible

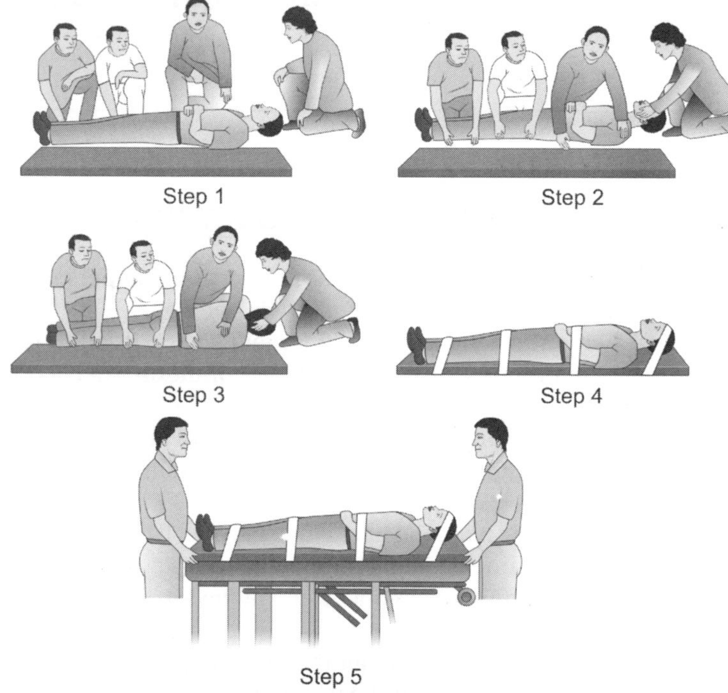

Fig. 1: A patient shifted by board

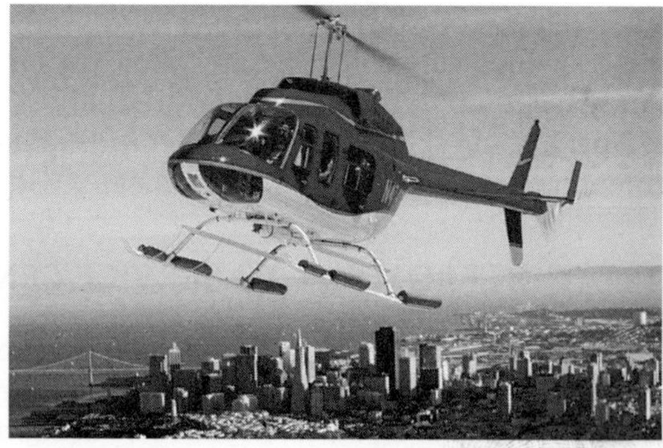

Fig. 2: Rapid transportation of patient by air from the site of injury to the Hospital

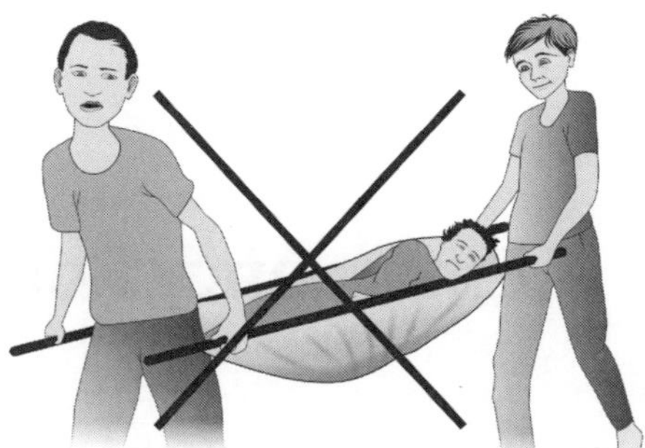

Fig. 3: A patient being carried with spine in flexion in a bed sheet

they should be air lifted by a helicopter to the hospital (Fig. 2). Person should never be carried in a bed sheet in a sagging position with the spine in flexion position (Fig. 3). Mass education through media to the society is essential in case the professional persons are not available for transportation.

Institution-based rehabilitation (IBR)—Concept is to transport patient with extrication board, collar, and belt by EMT.

Community-based rehabilitation (CBR)—Concept is the use of available resources, such as pillow as belt, shirt as collar.

14

Emergency Room Care

MEDICAL SCIENCE SERVICES

Apart from the usual trauma problems like bleeding, pain, distress (needs to be taken care); patients with spinal cord damage, face many problems of automatic regulation of heart rate, breathing, blood pressure, temperature, etc.

- Heart rate—Bradycardia may occur due to unopposed vagal activity (Thoracic sympathetic input may have been damaged.) Heart rate monitoring in ICU with administration of anticholinergic medications as prescribed
- Breathing—Problems depend on level and extent of injury.
  - C1-C4: Paralysis of diaphragm. A mechanical ventilator is required
  - C5-T6: Paralysis of intercostals (diaphragm is intact) needs respiratory support
  - T7-T12: Paralysis of abdominals with decreased function. Coughing is impaired.

Evaluate patient for the breathing rate and pattern, efforts, ability to cough, auscultate chest, and monitor SpO_2. Intubate or ventilate as per need. Oxygen supplement as needed. Tilt body in head up position. Ensure that the abdomen is not distended. Reference to physiotherapist to establish a regime of chest physio including assisted coughing.

BLOOD PRESSURE

Loss of automatic control results in vasodilatation and hypotension. This neurological stage lasts up to several weeks. Hypotension can lead to poor perfusion of edematous cord. Patient may need vasopressor drugs—noradrenaline or intravenous fluids to maintain BP (but excessive fluid can cause pulmonary edema).

TEMPERATURE

Inability to sweat, shiver, vasodilate, vasoconstrict to maintain body temperature. Adequate clothing, bedding in cold and fan, AC in hot atmosphere.

BLADDER

Reflex Bladder (Upper Motor)

Local reflex is intact. In T12 and above lesions, urination takes place by local reflex arc.

Flaccid Bladder (Lower Motor)

Local reflex is damaged. In T12 and below lesions, urination takes place by the overstretched detrusor. Irrespective of type of bladder, patient is put on indwelling catheter initially.

Urethral—Indwelling Foley's (flexible tube) catheter is inserted in the urethra which is kept there for a long time and changed in 2–4 week time. The catheter will have a balloon at the end that helps to keep in proper position. It continuously drains the bladder into the collection device, without the use of bladder contractions or co-ordinated action of sphincter control.

Suprapubic—Indwelling catheter is inserted into a bladder through a surgical opening in lower abdomen, just above pubic bone.

Benefits of Suprapubic is that (a) no damage to the urethra, (b) less likely for blockage as wider catheter is used, (c) easier to change and clean, (d) no damage to the sexual organs, (e) Easily reversible-opening gets healed within 1–2 days.

BOWEL

Reflex Bowel

Local reflex (Upper motor) is intact. In T12 and above lesions, with upper motor type, the ability to sense bowel may be lost. The reflexes and peristalsis movement moves the stool but the anal sphincter will remain tight and may need finger stimulation to open up and allow passage of stool.

Flaccid Bowel

Local reflex (Lower motor) is damaged. In T12 and below lesions with lower motor type, there may be damage to the defecation reflex which will relax the anal sphincter muscles. Reflexes that move the bowel is damaged. In this type, more attempts and manual removal of stool is needed. With inability of bowel movements, there may be impaction of stool.

All the medical emergencies are attended and person's vital signs are examined and necessary steps taken to make the medical condition of the patient stable. SCI patients have hypotension, hypoxia and anemia. SCI patients have decreased ability of spinal cord for autoregulation of its local blood flow, so the systemic blood flow and oxygenation needs to be maintained. Patient who can breathe when they come to the hospital, needs to be intubated, as cord edema progresses, respiration may become impaired. Mechanical ventilation relieves the muscle work of breathing and conserves the patient's energy during the emergent phase of the injury. An oral airway may be placed if a tracheostomy is unnecessary. Invasive hemodynamic monitoring is necessary in an intensive care unit postinjury. Foley's indwelling catheter is inserted through the urethra.

Necessary medications and injections are given to reduce pain, inflammations and other problems are also addressed, e.g. head injury or crush injury.

INFRASTRUCTURAL SUPPORT SERVICES AT REHABILITATION SET UP

Once the patient is examined and treated medically, it is advisable to transfer the patient to a rehab center for better prognosis. The rehab center must be well-equipped and have infrastructural support. One such center is Government Spine Institute, Civil Hospital, Ahmedabad, Gujarat, India. Government Civil Hospital is built in 110 acre land with extensive Medical education and service sections. It is a 2000 bed hospital with many specialty and superspeciality facilities. Medical and surgical emergencies are attended at Government Civil Hospital. Government Spine Institute Rehab set up with UG/PG-PT and UG-BPO programs.

ORTHOPEDIC SERVICES

For many SCI patients, orthopedic surgeon is in the front line for emergency measures with examination, evaluation and early management.

Diagnosis

The evaluation of the level and extent of lesion is done by clinical neurological examination of sensory, motor and reflex testing and with the help of X-ray, CT scan, myelogram, EMG-NCV and also with the help of lab tests. With American Spinal Injury Association (ASIA) or Frankel's scale complete or incomplete lesion with type is concluded.

Plan of Treatment

As per the merits of lesion, treatment is planned.

Nonsurgical (Noninvasive methods)

- Steroids: Methyl prednisolone sodium succinate (MPSS) is injected intravenously preferably within 8 hours of injury which reduces the inflammation and further damage to the cord
- Spine stabilization: Spine is stabilized or realigned by—
  - Immobilization for 6 weeks for cervical spine
  - Traction to reduce the dislocation of the spine (Fig. 1). Ortho injects Anzol to reduce pain, provide sedation. Patient is placed in prone position on traction table with a pillow under the tummy so as spine to come up. A tractive force of nearly 80 kg is applied. As the vertebrae are separated, physio/ortho will give manipulative force to reduce the dislocation
  - Continuous traction through skull bone with weights for 6 weeks in cases of cervical injury (Fig. 2).
  - External metal orthosis [sternal occipital mandibular immobilizer (SOMI) brace] for stable cervical injury (Fig. 3).
- Complete bed rest (No sitting or standing except log turning) for 3–4 weeks in stable thoracic and lumbar spine injury. Then after gradual graded tilting of spine (5 degrees every day to reach to upright within 3–4 weeks). For cervical spine injury with stable fracture 6 weeks immobilization is given with skull traction. Tilt table mobilization with gradual/graded tilting of 5 degrees each day after 6 weeks is started if condition is favorable.

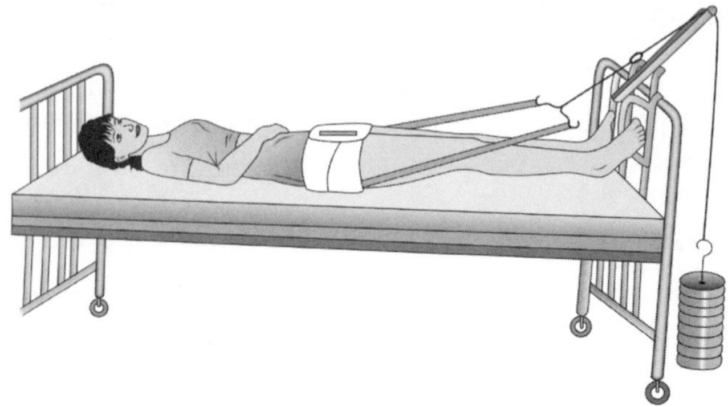

Fig. 1: Continuous lumbar spinal traction

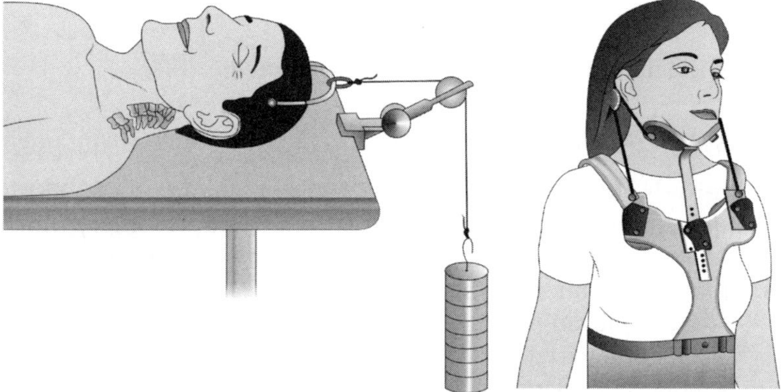

Fig. 2: Continuous cervical spinal traction

Fig. 3: Sternal occipital mandibular immobilizer (SOMI) Brace

Surgery

Spinal cord surgery is necessary in many cases to remove bone fragments, foreign object, herniated disk, fractured vertebra or anything that may be compressing the spinal cord. Surgery for the spinal fusion and spinal stabilization with internal fixations may also be needed.

- Spinal fusions: Surgical procedures to fuse or to join two or more vertebrae.
  - Anterior—The spine is operated from the front, disk from the lower part of the spine is removed and replaced it with a bone graft, desired result is that the two adjoining vertebrae to grow and fuse together into one solid bone

- Posterior—Same as anterior except that the approach is from back
- Lateral—Transforaminal fusion is done with the approach from side.

- Disc removal: Disc is removed which is compressing the spinal cord.
  - Cervical discectomy—Lumbar discectomy
  - Microdiscectomy—Minimally invasive surgery to remove ruptured disk.
- Surgical decompression: A small portion of the bone compressing over the nerve root is removed.
  - Foraminotomy—A foramen or opening from where the nerve roots come out of the spinal column is shaved and widened
  - Laminotomy—Partial removal of lamina or bony arches in the canal of spine
  - Laminectomy—Complete removal of the lamina
  - Corpectomy—Entire damaged vertebra is removed and replaced with bone graft.
- Laminoplasty—Lamina of both sides is cut open to create a space to relieve pressure on spinal cord.
  - Vertebroplasty/Kyphoplasty—A procedure to restore the vertebral height lost due to compression fracture.
- Spine stabilization with internal fixations:
  - Vertebral and pedicle fixation—In many unstable spine injuries, the pedicle is left intact even if the remaining vertebral segments are destroyed. The pedicle, which is the strongest part of vertebra, is a cylindrical, conical bone surrounding a small portion of inner cancellous bone. The pedicle connects the vertebral body to the posterior element
  - Since 1940s, the vertebral and pedicle fixations have evolved. Both the methods are designed to provide immediate stability and rigid immobilization of the spine without sacrificing the segmental motion of spine which is found in other conventional methods, e.g. Luque or Harrington rod fixation. The additional benefit of pedicle fixation is that it does not require intact lamina, facet joint or spinous processes
  - The history of vertebral screw fixation dates back to 1944. King first described the placement of screws (3/4" in women and 1" in men) parallel to the inferior border of lamina and perpendicular to the facet joints of lumbar vertebra

- Harrington rod fixation—Dr Paul Harrington in early 1960s revolutionized with his Harrington rod fixation in the correction of spinal deformity (Fig. 4). It was the first device to straighten and immobilize the spine from inside. The rod with the ratcheting mechanism is placed on the concavity side. One hook is attached at the top of the curve and other at the bottom of the curve. With ratcheting mechanism, the spine is stretched and straightened. As there are only two attachments, it is necessary to wear an external spinal brace postoperatively.
- Luque L rod fixation—Dr Eduardo Luque of Mexico City in early 1970s designed two flexible L-shaped rods which are placed on either side of the spine and are contoured to conform to the curve. The wires are threaded with sublaminar wiring at each segmental level. The wires are twisted around the rods which apply pressure over the rods that will straighten the spine. Since there are multiple levels of fixation patient does not have to wear an external brace as it is a case with Harrington rod. It has been widely adopted. It provides rigid fixation and allows early mobilization.
- Steffee pedicle and plate system—Dr Arthur Steffee in 1986 designed and described the use of plate with pedicle fixation which plays major role in thoracolumbar fixation. At present many pedicle screw and plate systems are available (Fig. 5).

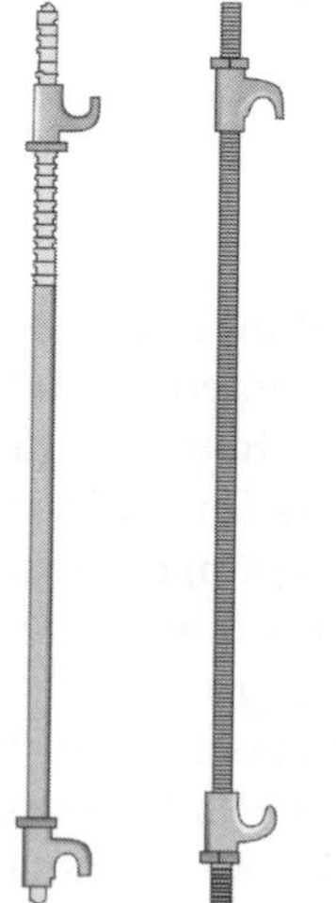

Fig. 4: Harrington rod fixation

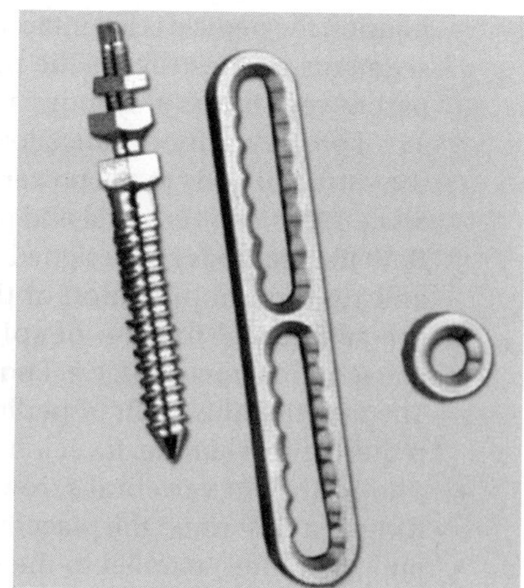

Fig. 5: Steffee fixation plate and screw

- Hartshill rectangle fixation—It is a modification of the Luque system of segmental spinal fixation. The rectangle is formed from a 3/16" stainless rod and incorporates a roof that allows fitting snugly against the lamina and provides the good rotational stability. The rectangle is secured to the spine by means of doubled 0.91 mm diameter stainless steel wires (Fig. 6).
- Moss Miami fixation—It is a versatile hook, rod and screw system utilizing poly axial screw technology and a patented dual closer mechanism offering 6 points of contacts with the rod. Moss Miami is available in titanium and stainless steel rod in a variety of diameters (Fig. 7).

Advantages of surgery

- It reduces the total rehabilitation period
- It reduces the complications of long bed ridden position
- It reduces the psychological problems
- It helps patient to channelize the brain energy for an early rehab
- It helps in neurological recovery.

After the immediate care of SCI with medical and orthopedic surgery—patient is first kept in ICU and after the stable medical condition, patient is transferred from intensive care unit (ICU) to the male/female wards.

Orthopedic surgeon examines and treats patients every day in the morning and evening. Neurologists, urologist, plastic surgeon are consulted, if there is a need.

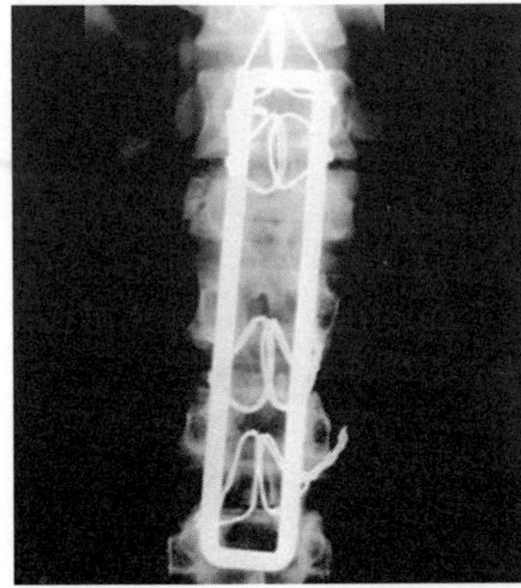

Fig. 6: Hartshill rectangle fixation

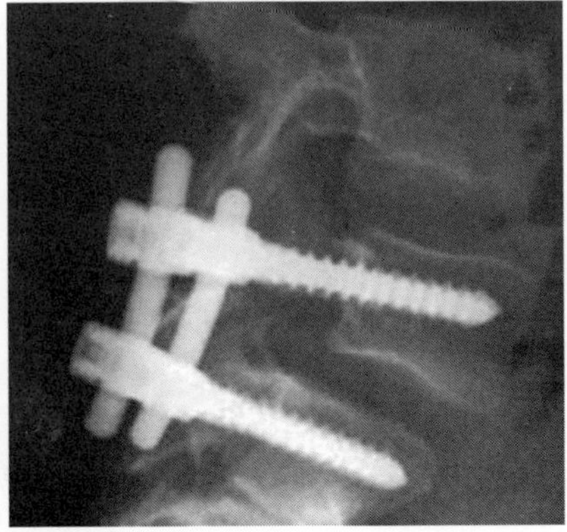

Fig. 7: Moss Miami pedicle screw fixation

Orthopedics for Complications

Contractures: a) Serial plaster casting, b) Surgical soft tissue release (e.g. Tendo achilles for equinus, hip and knee flexor release for flexion contractures, joint replacement for hip, etc.)

Pressure sores: Bed sore debridement, skin grafting.

Steroid (Kenakort) injections to reduce the complications and to improve function. (A paper presented by Mrs Yagna Shukla, Mrs Anjali Bhise and Professor Dr Prabhakar)

Kenakort is injected in the epidural space under aseptic precautions.

Effects:

- Spasticity reduction 33%
- Voluntary control improvement 16%
- Withdrawals reductions >50% a) ADL improvement >60% b) In ROM resistance is reduced

15

Nursing Services

Of all rehab team members, nursing team has the maximum contact time with SCI patients, providing services for 24 hours in three shifts. They are in survival and settlement phases. Matron is the head of nursing team of all the wards. Every ward has in-charge sister, clinical sisters and students. Many SCI setups realize that nurses and related professionals need additional knowledge and skills for the complex care and needs of SCI rehab program.

- Nursing services: Primary services (Fig. 1)
  - To provide prescribed medicines
  - Inject medicines
  - Do dressing of the wound
  - Bladder and bowel care
  - Monitoring of vital signs
  - Call the consultants
  - Coordination of medical and rehab services
  - Maintaining treatment records.

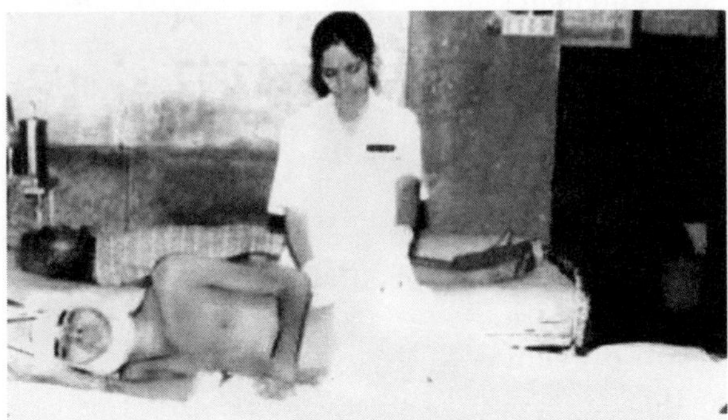

Fig. 1: SCI patient management by Nurse

- Nursing services: Other important services are:
  - Food and fluid services
  - Transportation to and from appointments
  - Light housekeeping
  - Patient's personal hygiene
  - Care of bed, instruments and gadgets used.

Skin care: SCI patients have sensory loss. Decubitus ulcers (pressure sores, bed sores) are very common. Special program is set for them.

To keep the cloth and bed sheets dry and creaseless. (SCI have possibility of bladder, bowel accidents, consequently soiling clothes and bed sheets).

Skin Inspection: Skin needs to be inspected. Patients are also taught how to see paralyzed parts with a long handled mirror.

Wet skin is cleaned with spirit and kept dry with talcum powder. Deodorant is sprayed to mask the foul odor. Skin is protected from hot and sharp objects.

PRESSURE SORE PREVENTION

Our brain has set weight relieving programs. We do not remain in one position or posture constantly and change it frequently automatically-even during sleep we change our sleep positions. SCI patients are at a disadvantage doubly, they neither have sensory feedback, nor do they have motor ability to move paralyzed parts. Over and above, if the skin is wet, it starts breaking easily. After 2 hours of constant pressure with one position on the skin, it starts showing the changes of pressure sores hence it is utmost important to properly take care of pressure sores so as to prevent them (Fig. 2).

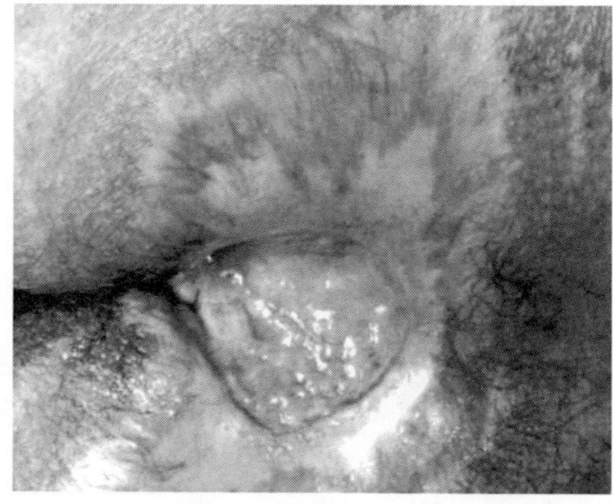

Fig. 2: Pressure sore over the sacral region just above the gluteal fold in a patient with paraplegia

Two hourly regime of log turning: With the help of three persons, the whole body (like a log-like a whole wooden block) is turned to right or left side or to prone position, every two hourly. In log turning, the spine is kept straight to avoid any stress or strain to the injured cord.

There are different types of beds: Beds with removable side bars, facility to raise the upper or lower part as per need, bed with soft mattresses, three piece bed, water bed, air rippling bed—electrically operated, roto rest oscillating bed—a mechanical-electrically operated bed to turn the patient's position (supine to prone and back).

Positioning of Body

Paralyzed parts have a tendency of developing soft tissue tightness which later on become contracture (Tightness of soft tissues can be lengthened to its full length passively whereas the contractures cannot be lengthened). The limbs are placed in "Functional positions" (so that even if the contracture takes place, patient can perform functions with available range). Body part positioning is maintained with the help of pillows, sandbags, splints.

BEDSORE/PRESSURE ULCER (DECUBITUS ULCER-PRESSURE SORE) MANAGEMENT

Education of patient, families, and healthcare providers is the key to a proactive program of prevention and timely interventions from a multidisciplinary approach.

Significance/Impact of the Problem

- Pressure sore (PS) incidence is associated with an increased morbidity and mortality, nearly 70% die within 6 months (Brown 2003)
- PS incidence increases long-term care and cost (LTC) (Hom et al. 2004)
- Skin and wound allegations are second leading litigation in LTC (Chizen)
- They are very painful thus causing patients a great deal of suffering
- Because of the foul odor, they deprive patient for social participation
- An ulcer that heals, forms scar tissue, lacks the original elasticity, likely to ulcerate again and again

- Like any other complication, it deprives patient, from rehab program
- Abuse to the hospital staff for neglect, malpractice.

Pressure ulcer is caused by forces—sustain position, friction and shearing that block the flow of blood to the skin leading to tear and ulceration. They generally develop above tail bone, buttocks, trochanters, heels, scapula and elbows.

Sign and Symptoms

Many patients do not know that they have pressure ulcer. It is first noticed by the family members/nurses/rehab professionals. It is noticed while bathing, clothing, bedding with presence of skin discoloration and due to foul odor and pain.

Contributing factors:

- Intrinsic factors: Malnutrition, dehydration, impaired mobility, sensory loss, chronic conditions, infections, advance age, diabetes.
- External factors: Pressure, friction, shear, moisture, incontinence.

Prevention (An ounce of prevention is worth a pound of cure):

- Provide soft, smooth-support surface
- Regular reposition every 2 hours
- Use pillows or positioning boot
- Use pillows between knees in side-lying
- Avoid friction—a mechanical force exerted when skin is dragged on a coarse surface. Shear is the mechanical force caused by the interplay of gravity and friction which cause angulation and stretching of blood vessels, causing thrombosis and cellular death. This manifest as necrosis and undermining of deepest layers. Use draw sheets for repositioning, proper transfer techniques to avoid frictions and shear forces
- Apply emollient ointment to intact skin for softening and to keep skin pliable
- If skin is red or denuded, use a paste
- Use proper incontinence disposals
- Control diabetes
- Avoid cold, caffeine, narcotics.

ASSESSMENT OF BED SORE

Wound assessment is done weekly to drive decisions.

General Assessment

- Systemic factors: Etiology, duration, decreased oxygenation or perfusion of wound, comorbid conditions, medications and host infection of the patient
- Psychological factors: Patient's knowledge deficits, cultural beliefs, financial constrain, social support, impaired accessibility to resources
- Location: Body part with a nearest bony prominence or landmark. Class/Stage is defined by the "National Pressure Ulcer Advisory Panel (NPUAP)"
- Risk factors: Barden and Norton scales are developed to assess the risk factors of age, fever, poor protein intact, sensory perception, moisture, activity, mobility, friction and shear forces
- Stages: Originally, there were four stages but from 2007, there are now six stages.
    1. Stage I—Intact skin with nonblanchable redness of a localized area, usually over a bony prominence. Dark pigmented skin, may look purple and may not have visible blanching; its color, skin is warmer, may differ from the surrounding area
    2. Stage II—Partial thickness loss of dermis presenting as a shallow open ulcer with a red/pink wound bed, without slough. May also present as an intact or open/ruptured serum filled blister
    3. Stage III—Full thickness skin loss, subcutaneous fat may be visible but bone, tendon or muscle is not exposed. Slough may be present but does not obscure the depth of tissue loss. May include undermining tunneling
    4. Stage IV—Full thickness skin loss with exposed bone, tendon, muscle. Slough or Eschar may be present on some parts of the wound bed often include tunneling and undermining
    5. Stage V—Unstageable—full thickness tissue loss in which the base of the ulcer is covered by slough (yellow, tan, gray, green or brown) and/or eschar (tan, brown, black) in the wound bed
    6. Stage VI—Suspected deep tissue injury—purple or maroon localized area of discolored intact skin or blood-filled blister due to damage of underlying soft tissue from pressure and/or shear.

The area may be preceded by the tissue that is painful, firm, mushy, boggy, warmer or cooler as compared to adjacent tissue.

Class

- Partial thickness wound (PTW)—damage to epidermis and/or dermis only
- Full thickness wound (FTW)—damage to subcutaneous layer or deeper.

Size Measurement

- Length—from top edge to bottom edge at longest point
- Width—from edge-to-edge perpendicular to the length at widest point
- Depth—straight in, perpendicular to the base at deepest point.

Undermining-Tunneling

- Using the clock concept (12 o'clock is in the direction of the patient's head and 6 o'clock is towards the feet)
- Where does it starts and where does it end (clockwise direction)
- Tunnel depth at its deepest point
- Location of deepest point.

Wound Bed/Base Assessment

- Necrosis/eschar—black, brown devitalized tissue, adhered to wound bed or edges
- Slough—soft, moist, avascular tissue that adhered to the wound bed in string or thick clumps—may be white, yellow, tan or green
- Granulation—Pink/red moist tissue comprised of new blood vessels, collagen fiber and fibroblasts. Typically, the surface is shiny and moist with granular appearance
- Epithelium—New pink and shiny tissue/skin that grows in from the edges or as an islands on the wound surface.

Exudates

Amount

- None: Base and dressing dry
- Slight: Small amount in the center of dressing
- Moderate: Contained within the dressing
- Copious: Extends beyond dressing onto clothing or bed linen.

Type

- Serous: Thin, watery, clear or straw colored
- Serosanguinous: Thin, pale, red to pink
- Purulent: Thick, opaque, tan, yellow to green and may have an offensive odor.

Odor

- Most wounds have an odor. Extreme malodor with purulent exudate is with infection.

Edge/Perimeter

- Edge: Approximated, rolled, calloused
- Peri wound skin: Indurated, erythematous, macerated, healthy
- Presence of excoriation, denudement, erosion, papules, pastures or other lesions
- Induration: Abnormal hardening of the tissue caused by consolidation of edema, this may be a sign of underlying infection
- Erythema: Redness of surrounding tissue may be normal in the inflammatory stage of healing. However, if accompanied by an increase in temperature of tissue, exudates or pain may also be a sign of an infection
- Maceration: Caused by excessive moisture, tissue loses, its pigmentation (appears lucid or turns white) and becomes soft and friable.

Infection Signs and Symptoms

- Redness, warmth and induration of adjacent tissues
- Pain or tenderness
- Dysmorphic and/or friable granulation
- Unusual odor
- Purulent exudates
- Systemic signs (fever, chills, sweats).

Culture Testing

- It is done when signs of infection are present or when clean wound fails to heal
- Semiquantitative swab collection is acceptable
- Quantitative biopsy is "gold standard" but expensive and invasive.

Physical Examination

- Edema: Extent and persistence of pitting
- Color changes: Dependent rubor (purple-red discoloration) or elevation pallor (paling of the skin when leg is raised to a 60 degrees angle for 15–60 seconds)
- Distal pulse: Amplitude on palpation
- Neuropathy: Skin changes (dryness, cracking), structural abnormalities, loss of protective sensation.

Diagnostic Tests

- Ankle-Brachial index: Comparison of perfusion pressure
- Pulse volume recording: Perfusion volume
- Doppler wave forms: single vessel flow
- Duplex imaging-ultrasound imaging for venous disease (also test for DVT)
- Transcutaneous oxygen pressure ($TcpO_2$).

Wound Healing

The healing process depends on stage. Stage I and II and partial thickness heal by tissue regeneration. Stage III and IV and full thickness heal by scar formation and contraction (need skin grafting). Data indicate a 20% reduction in wound size over 2 weeks is a reliable predictive indicator of healing.

- Inflammatory phase
  - 0–3 days
  - Hemostasis (bleeding stops)
  - Inflammation (redness, swelling, warmth, pain may be present)
  - Phagocytosis (WBC's engulf bacteria and foreign debris).
- Proliferation phase
  - 3–21 days
  - Angiogenesis (new blood vessels develop)
  - Collagen synthesis (protein fibers)
  - Granulation formation
  - Epithelialization
  - Contraction.
- Maturation phase
  - 21 days–2 years
  - Reorganization of collagen
  - Tensile strength improves (80%).

Optimization of Wound Environment

- Manage comorbid conditions:
  - Optimize cardiovascular and pulmonary functions
  - Support tissue oxygenation
  - Maintain blood glucose level.
- Adequate nutrition and hydration:
  - Encourage protein, calorie dense food and fluid
  - Monitor intake, weight, skin turgor.
- Eliminate or minimize pain:
  - Treat the cause, e.g. infection medicines
  - Psychosocial, spiritual, cultural sensitive support
  - Gentle dressing removal.

Cleansing of Wound

- Normal saline is recommended solution
- Cavity, tunnels may be irrigated
- Force, pressure to remove debris without harming healthy tissue.

Protecting Wound and Periwound Skin

- Barrier products to protect from adhesives and moisture
- Change dressings at appropriate intervals to avoid pooling of exudates.

Prevent and manage infection: Critical colonization can result in failure to heal, poor quality tissue, increase friability.

Debridement: Removal of Nonviable Tissue

Contraindications

- Dry stable heel eschar
- Ischemic wounds with dry gangrene
- Coagulation disorder.

Types of Debridement

- Autolytic debridement
  - Lysis of necrotic tissue by the body's white blood cells and enzymes
  - Leaves healthy tissue intact
  - Natural physiological process in moist atmosphere.

- Chemical debridement
  - Collagenase (Santyl)
  - Papain with urea (Ethezyme)
  - Denaturing agents—Sodium hydrochlorite (Clorpactin) a nonselective method.
- Mechanical debridement
  - Wet to dry dressing (not recommended as it is nonselective, causes repeated trauma and is painful)
  - Whirlpool (risk of cross contamination and contraindicated for some wounds, such as venous stasis)
  - Pulse lavage (requires skill, rigorous infection control precautions and cost prohibitive).
- Sharp surgical debridement
  - Sequential removal of avascular tissue, using sterile scalpel and mouse-tooth forceps
  - Premedicate if wound is painful
  - Avoid local anesthesia.

How can a physiotherapist help in pressure sore ulcer?

Wound care is a part of physiotherapy practice from the beginning.

- Train the family and caretakers: PT and OT together train one and all how to position and reposition, transfer on bed, wheel chair, toilet seat, bedside commode, chair
  - Frequent small position change by patient is faster, easier, safer
  - A small pillow behind the shoulder or hip alters position without having to move entire body
  - Head of bed at 30 degrees or less to avoid sliding body down with shear
  - Have the patient assist in moving by using overhead "trapeze bar"
  - Patient on chair must form habit to do weight transfers every 15 minutes by chair pushups, leaning forward, side to side, backward (Leaning forward is easiest and effective).
- Improve strength: Upper limbs are strengthened by "Pull up-Push up" exercises.
- Habit to inspect skin visually, daily with a long handle mirror. Palpation—press the vulnerable skin with finger tip. Initially skin will become pale but within 2–3 seconds the skin color will be same as surrounding skin, indicates good circulation
- Habit formation: Patients "must develop habit" to shift body weight or reposition

- Educate patient/care giver about signs to look for the wound healing process
- Modification of sitting/sleeping surfaces to reduce the pressure
- Support surface: There is no mattress that will eliminate pressure and relieve. Patient, clinician or care taker must reposition the patient.

PT-Electro and Therapeutic measures

- Soft tissue mobilization: The surrounding skin is moved gently with hands to help venous return and to improve oxygenation through improved circulation
- Infrared radiation: Close wound and irradiate surrounding skin with infrared rays to provide mild heat to increase blood circulation
- Ultraviolet (Type B-Short wavelength—UVR from fluorescent tube UVR lamp): Treatment dosage—a) Floor-E4 dose, b) Wall-E3 dose c) Base-E2 dose.
  - Bactericidal (Bacteria destruction)—Short wavelength UVR has enough energy to damage chemical bonds in DNA molecule of bacteria, which are very stable under most conditions
  - Epithelialization—UVR increases epithelial proliferation
  - Size—UVR produces reduction in both the surface area and volume of the ulcer.
- LASER (Light amplification by stimulated emission of radiation): Various types of LASER are used for diagnosis, treatment and therapy (Fig. 3).
  - Gas lasers—(HeNe) Helium-Neon, Carbon dioxide, Argon-ion
  - Chemical—Hydrogen fluoride, ethylene in nitrogen
  - Trifluoride-Excimer—Powered by an electric discharge
  - Solid state use crystalline or glass rod-ruby laser
  - Titanium-doped sapphire.
- Electrical stimulations: Low amplitude monophasic direct currents >1 second or biphasic pulsed currents are used to stimulate the tissues

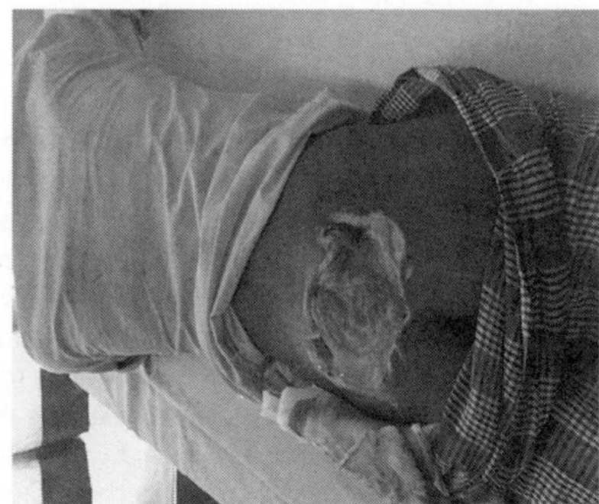

Fig. 3: LASER therapy for pressure sore

- Monophasic current is a direct continuous unidirectional flow of current is used as the wound have negative polarity compared to the surrounding skin. The current facilitates phagocytosis and autolysis in the inflammatory stage. Current attracts the electrically charged cells, such as leukocytes and neutrophils and stimulates the proliferation and activity of fibroblasts to increase collagen synthesis. Negative electrode should be used selected initially if the wound is infected with the organism sensitive to cathodal stimulation, e.g. *E. coli* and *P. aeruginosa*. Positive pole is more beneficial if the wound is infected with bacteria, e.g. *S. aureus*.

- Iontophoresis: Gentamicin iontophoresis, Zinc (Zinc Oxide) iontophoresis
- Whirlpool bath: Patient's pressure sore part is immersed in the water with disinfectant in the Whirlpool tub. The whirling of the water will have mechanical effect for debridement of dead and infected tissues also the mechanical force of the water will improve blood circulation and will improve the epithelialization.

Onigbinde AT, Olafimihan KF, Ojoawo A, Mothabeng J, Ogundiran OO. Management of Decubitus Ulcer using Gentamycin Sulphate Iontophoresis—A Case Study. The Internet Journal of Allied Health Sciences and Practice. Jan 2011. Volume 9 Number 1.

Abstract:

Most infective organisms have developed resistance against antibiotics. There is need to find other means to deliver antibiotics locally. There appears to be limited studies on the use of gentamicin sulfate iontophoresis in wound management. The participant in this study was a subject diagnosed with mild head injury secondary to motor vehicle accident who later developed a unilateral pressure sore on the left gluteal region. The subject received 15-minutes of gentamicin sulfate iontophoresis (Interrupted Direct Current) 3 times a week for 5 weeks. The case report showed that there was a 65.7% reduction in wound surface area of the decubitus ulcer at the end of five weeks. Also, bacterial growth reduced from very heavy growth to scanty growth at the end of the 5th week. This report suggested that gentamicin sulfate ointment iontophoresis as adjunct with traditional saline-wet-to-moist (WM) wound dressing had an effect in healing the decubitus ulcer of the participant used in this study.

BLADDER CARE

Initially, patient is on indwelling continuous catheter. With continuous catheterization, detrusor-bladder muscle does not get stretch nor there is a chance for bladder to contract. To avoid shrinkage of bladder and a chance for bladder to contract, intermittent clamping regime is adopted. The clamp is released at regular interval to void urine and avoid over distention.

Indwelling catheter becomes a hurdle for PT/OT and rehab programs; also there are hazards of it. (Urethritis, urethral fistula, stricture urethra, purulent cystitis, renal failure, Delay in bladder recovery, Difficult to know about the bladder recovery, scrotal abscess) To avoid these problems of continuous catheterization, in 1943 Riches, started with removal of continuous catheter and insertion of catheter only for voiding of urine. In late 1940s, when antibiotics became available, Guttmann and Frenkel suggested "Aseptic intermittent catheterization."

Self-intermittent catheterization: Lepides et al. in 1971 introduced the concept of clean, self-intermittent catheterization, which is simple and safe.

Technique

Either latex or PVC, 14F catheter is used. Patient or a relative is instructed to clean the genital with water and soap. Then wash the hands and the catheter with soap and water, three times. Liquid paraffin is applied on catheter without drying. Patient or care taker inserts the catheter in the urethra gently.

Male: Hold glans penis with left thumb and index finger, now with right hand slowly and smoothly insert the catheter in urethra, till urine drainage starts.

Female: Spread the labia with left thumb and index finger. With the tactile sensation of right hand, the urethral opening is located and reassured repeatedly. Insert catheter slowly and smoothly till urine drainage starts. (Dr Sarla Bhatt, Dr Dilip Patel presented a scientific paper on "Self-catheterization in the national Conference of Physiotherapy held at Ahmedabad, Gujarat, India in 1985).

BOWEL CARE

Patients are trained for taking care of bowel as per the level of lesion and the type of bowel. Constipation is avoided which can lead to impaction. Adequate fluid and fiber diet is given for smooth motion. If needed, liquid paraffin is given or suppository is placed. Fecal impaction is removed with gloved fingers.

16

Physiotherapy in the Intensive Care Unit

On admission, Physios appear in intensive care unit (ICU). Since breathing is controlled by autonomic nervous system (ANS) in upper spinal cord, spinal cord injury (SCI) patients with upper cord lesions face difficulty in breathing. Thanks to recent medical technology which enables a patient to breathe with assistance of devices (diaphragm pacemaker, manual-mechanical ventilators) medications and physiotherapy. SCI is susceptible to pneumonia, collapsed lungs (atelectasis), hence careful and continuous monitoring is required. For the use of a ventilator a tube (tracheostomy—a surgical opening in the neck or endotracheal tube in which a tube is entered through the natural mouth or nose opening to the tracheal airway) or mask is used.

In ICU—Physio does evaluation and assessment of patient with inspection, palpation, percussion, auscultation, pulmonary function test (PFT) and plans program accordingly.

- Inspection/Observation: Breath pattern—regular or deep, distressed, labored, use of accessory muscles. Color of skin, lips and nail bed (Blue is bad—Cyanosis)
  - Position of patient—Pulmonary dysfunction-sit upright
  - Distress—lean forward hands on knees, tri-pod position in emphysema, pursed lip breathing—emphysema, asthma
  - Ability to speak—fewer words per breath worse the problem
  - Abdominal wall moving inward in inspiration due to flattened diaphragm in emphysema
  - Chest deformity—pectus excavatum—concave lower sternum, barrel chest—increased anterior posterior diameter with flat diaphragm in emphysema.
- Palpation provides primary (basic) information about lung diseases

- Accentuating chest excursion—rub hands, make them warm and place on patient's back with thumb pointed towards spine. When patient takes deep breath, the hands should lift symmetrically normally. The hand on affected side lifts to a lesser degree suggests air or fluid-filled pleural space
- Tactile fremitus—place your hands from ulnar sides firmly on either side of back. Ask patient to say the words "ninety nine". A vibratory sound is transmitted to the hands which is a normal fremitus. It is a subtle finding and not just primary
- Lung consolidation—lung filled with fluid or tissue, e.g. pneumonia, fremitus becomes more pronounced
- Pleural effusion—the fremitus is decreased.

• Percussion requires fine skillful movement of right wrist, hammering right middle fingertip on left middle finger which is placed on chest or back and sensitive ear to hear.
  - Normal lung—resonant note.
  - Fluid in the cavity (Pleural effusion) or infiltration of white cells and bacteria (pneumonia) makes dull sound
  - Air trapping (emphysema or pneumothorax) hyperresonant-drum like sound.
• Auscultation: (Latin verb—auscultate means to listen) Listening of abnormal body sounds—lungs, heart, blood vessels, bowel, fetus, joints for its frequency, intensity, duration and quality for diagnosis.

  Auscultation requires experience, listening skill, fine stethoscope.
  - Immediate—unaided, directly with ears, e.g. grating of a moving joint
  - Mediate—use of an instrument, e.g. Stethoscope Breath sounds:
    - Bronchial, bronchovesicular, vesicular—breathing with normal tidal volume
    - Wheeze—whistling noises on expiration when air is forced out from narrowed airways by bronchoconstriction, secretions, mucosal edema (emphysema, asthma)
    - Stridor—wheezing is heard only on inspiration due to obstruction at trachea
    - Rales—(a.k.a. Crackles) scratchy sounds (rubbing strands of hair together close to ear) due to fluid within alveolar and interstitial spaces, e.g. Pulmonary edema. In pneumonia, sound is restricted in alveolar filling. In

pulmonary fibrosis, distinct, diffuse, dry sounds like crackles (separating Velcro) is heard
- Tubular or bronchial breath sounds in dense consolidation of lung parenchyma, transmission of a large central airway noises [similar to snorkel sound (a tube for swimmer to breathe with face in water)]
- Egophony—auscultation in consolidated involved lobe and patient is asked to say "eee", it is detected as a nasal sound "aaa"
- Ronchi—secretions, mucous in larger airways produce gurgling type noise like sucking last bits of milk shake with a straw.

Computer-aided electronic stethoscope and Auscultogram can help to record findings for teaching and telemedicine (remote diagnosis and treatment). Doppler auscultation is sensitive than simple auscultation.

PULMONARY FUNCTION TEST

- A simple way to measure lung capacity is to measure chest expansion with a measure tape at the end of inspiration (2–2.5 inches expansion at xiphisternum)
- Pulse oximeter: A device which continuously measures heart rate and oxygen saturation in blood. Shortness of breath is a sign of cardiac or pulmonary dysfunction on exercises and exertion
- Spirometer: In 1621, Dr Borelli assembled a cylindrical tube partially filled with water with an open water source entering the bottom of the cylinder. He occluded his nostrils, inhaled through an opening at the top of the cylinder and measured the volume of air displaced by water.

  Present electronic spirometer compute airflow rate and volume, using ultrasonic transducer or pressure difference channels with accuracy by eliminating the momentum and resistance errors of moving parts.

  Following are the findings of the spirometry:
  - Total lung capacity (TLC)—Volume of air in lungs on maximum inflation VC+RV
  - Vital capacity (VC)—Volume of max air breathed out after deepest inhalation
  - Reserve volume (RV)—Volume of air remaining in lungs after maximum exhalation

- Tidal volume (TV)—Volume of air moving in and out of lungs at rest (Approx 500 mL)
- Expiratory reserved volume (ERV)—Volume of air exhaled from the end of resting expiration
- Inspiratory reserved volume (IRV)—Volume of air inspired from the end of resting inspiration
- Inspiratory capacity (IC)—Volume of air IRV + TV
- Inspiratory vital capacity (IVC)—Volume of maximum air inhaled from maximum expiration
- Functional residual capacity (FRC)—Volume of air in lungs at the end of expiration
- Forced expiratory volume (FEV1)—Volume of air forced out in first second.
- Forced vital capacity (FVC)—Vital capacity from a forced maximum expiratory effort.
- Peak expiratory flow (PEF)—Peak level of expiration.
- FiO_2—Fraction (%) of inspired oxygen.

Total lung capacity (TLC), functional residual capacity (FRC), residual volume (RV) are increased (too much air and take longer time to empty) in obstructive lung diseases (There is increased airway resistance due to bronchospasm with early closer of airways, resulting in air trapping, e.g. emphysema, asthma, chronic bronchitis, cystic fibrosis) and TLC, FRC, RV are decreased in restrictive lung diseases (Lungs inflation is restricted due to deformity kyphoscoliosis, paralysis of muscles, pneumonia, pleural effusion, radiation fibrosis).

PHYSIO TREATMENT IN INTENSIVE CARE UNIT

Physiotherapists follow scientific principles with programs as per "ABC" rule to treat patient (Figs 1A and B).

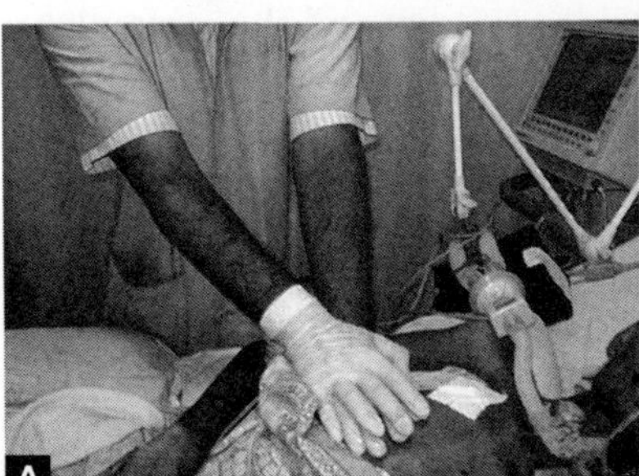

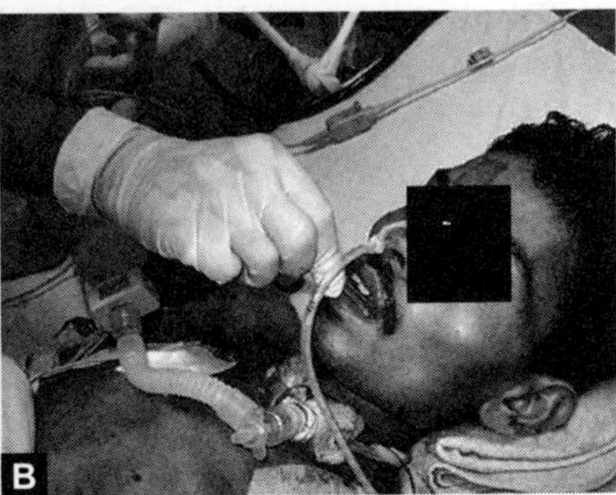

Figs 1A and B: Physiotherapy management in ICU—A patient receiving vibration manipulations (A) followed by suction (B)

"A" Airway Clearance

If there is blockage due to collections of secretions, suction is carried out or "postural drainage" is done with available positions and airway is cleared.

Postural Drainage

Patient should be well hydrated with water. Find out the possible position for the segment to remain upper most so as the gravity assists the drainage and oxygenation. After 15–20 minutes of gravity dependent position, agility exercises are done (deep breathing, unaffected body parts movements) also hacking, clapping tapotements are carried out to loosen the sputum. After that patient does huffing and coughing to remove the secretions and sputum. It is best done in the morning (secretions accumulate in the night), 2 hours after meals to avoid gastroesophageal reflux.

Huffing

Following a deep inhalation, patient attempts short frequent exhalation by contracting abdominal muscles and saying "ha ha ha". The glottis remains open. The secretion gets dislodged and it moves from the peripheral to central airway.

Coughing

Patient preferably sits in an upright position (or in an available position). Cough generation is produced by large inspiration volume, patient holds breath for several seconds with closed glottis, allows intrathoracic pressure to build up, patient leans forward (or turns head to one side if patient is lying) and with a sudden and sharp expulsive expiration produced by intercostals (thoracic roots) and abdominals (T4-L1), patient opens glottis and exhales and expels sputum and secretions in a bowl filled with disinfectant (or a bowl with sand). Cough is important for airway clearance, prevention of respiratory tract infection and atelectasis (collapsed lungs). Respiratory system has other roles to play—gaseous exchange, speaking and posture-related activities.

Active cycles of breathing technique (ACBT) to clear the secretions. Breath control: Breath control is used to relax the airways and relieve the symptoms of sensitive airways for tightness and wheeze after coughing. Rest one hand on stomach, relax your shoulder girdle. Breathe in slowly, smoothly. Your hand should rise up. Hold for 3–4 seconds, breath out gently and quietly. Your hand will fall towards spine. Generally, 3 or 4 repetitions are performed but more in breathlessness.

Thoracic expansion exercise: This will help air to get behind the stuck sputum. Rest and relax your upper chest, breathe in slowly, smoothly and deeply. Breath-out gently, quietly for a prolonged period. Do not force out air. Do it 3–4 times, if you feel lightheaded go back to relaxed breathing.

Forced expiratory technique: Huffing to loosen secretions and to take it from periphery to central airways and then do coughing to expel out sputum. If you do not produce cough in 1–2 coughs, repeat the cycle.

"B" Breathing

Artificial Breathing Devices

Manual ventilators:

Artificial manual breathing unit (AMBU) bag (AMBU Resuscitator—AR) is the most simple, safe, cheap unit. Air is pushed through the connecting tube in the lungs by squeezing bag with a hand, on release the air will come out. AR does not allow for detection of patient's spontaneous ventilation. Nowadays, AR is modified by incorporating an incentive spirometer which allows for the detection and volume assessment of patient's spontaneous breathing.

Anesthesia bag: A soft rubber bag used as part of a gas flow system to monitor and control the patient's breathing. This supple bag is less fatiguing to the hands of the operator.

Mechanical ventilator:

It requires electric power supply—battery or wall outlet.

Negative pressure: The iron lung was first developed in 1929. Patient is placed in a large elongated iron tank. The neck and head is outside the tank in the atmospheric ambient air. By means of a mechanical pump, the air from the tank is withdrawn which creates a negative pressure in the tank which expands lungs allowing ambient air to flow in the lungs. As the vacuum is released, elastic recoil of chest and lungs leads to passive exhalation.

Positive pressure: The modern positive pressure ventilators are mainly based on developments by the military during World War

II to supply oxygen to fighter pilots in high altitudes. They work by increasing the patient's airway pressure through an endotracheal tube or a tracheostomy tube. The positive pressure allows the air to flow into the airway until the ventilator breath is terminated, subsequently the airway pressure drops to zero and the elastic recoil of the chest and lungs push out the tidal volume.

Diaphragm pace maker: A device which is surgically implanted to help with breathing by stimulating phrenic nerve, using electrical stimulations. A ventilator is likely to be required.

Girder/Abdominal binders are used to prevent abdominal contents falling forward in an upright posture. They are used in subjects with abdominal weakness (lesions T6 and-above). In tetraplegia, binders help to increase vital capacity and decrease in FRC.

SCI at most levels affects innervation of abdominals which affects the ability to forcefully contract abdominals during coughing to clear the secretions.

Abdominals (mainly transverse abdominis) play important role in breathing and coughing. Place your hand on lower abdomen, ask patient to breathe out and at the end of expiration, patient gives extra efforts to tighten abdomen to push out air.

The strong abdominals will push the viscera inside and the diaphragm will go up. During this relaxed-resting position, the aperture (Vena cava) in the diaphragm is wide open which allows maximum blood to go back to heart, better stroke volume, better gaseous exchange in lungs and thereby better nutrition to tissue with better oxygenated blood to body and brain.

Active Breathing Devices

Balloon blowing: Patient will blow air in the balloon. This will strengthen the respiratory muscles and it will also increase the vital capacity. Prolonged breathing out will help to remove residual air from the lungs.

Incentive (motivational) spirometer: A simple device with three tubes with small balls inside the tubes. It is connected with an air blowing/air sucking pipe (Fig. 2).

Inspiration—Patient sucks air from the pipe which is connected to the device. The balls in the tube will go up. With less effort one ball will go up, with more efforts 2nd...3rd...ball will go up and is made to hold approx 10 seconds. Aim is not the number of balls going up, but

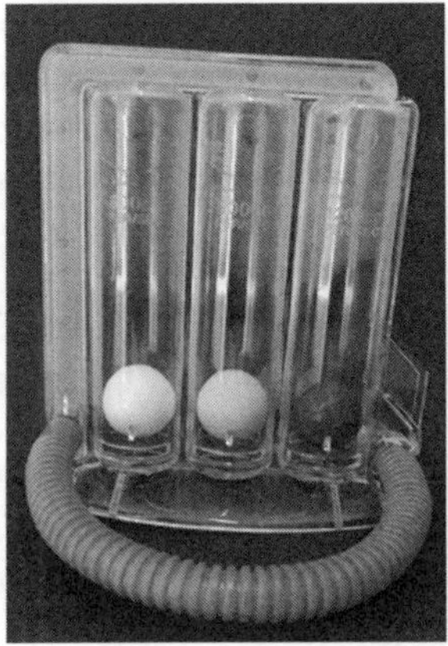
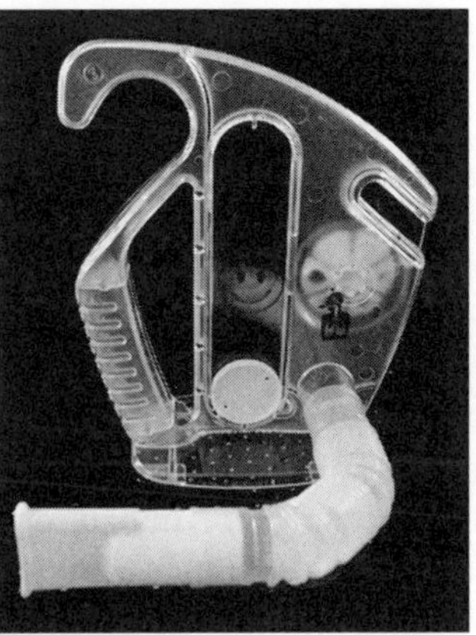

Fig. 2: Incentive spirometer (by inhaling through the tube, the ball(s) in the device are lifted up giving visual feedback

how much time he is able to maintain the ball up. This will increase the inspirational capacity. Expiration—Now reverse the device and blow air in the pipe. As above stated, the balls will go up one by one. This will increase the expiration capacity.

Breathing Techniques

Physios pay special attention for hypertrophy of the remaining muscles individually and in a group and teach, train and test patients, how to use different techniques of breathing and coughing. The techniques are explained and then demonstrated or specific video is shown.

Diaphragmatic breathing: Patient takes air in lower lobes and abdomen will go up. Patient's or professional's hands on abdominals, will give a push during expiration.

Segmental breathing: Patient slowly inspires and clinician/care taker, resist it maximally (but allows the inspiration to take place) with hand on the selected segment. During expiration, the same hand provides pressure to expel maximum air from the segment.

Costal breathing: Patient sits in front of a big mirror [(for a mirror biofeedback-visual cueing)(tactile cueing is given by hand placements)(Auditory cueing is given by sharp and specific command, e.g. inspire and lift your chest cage)]. During inspiration, patient consciously lifts the chest wall with visual, tactile, auditory feedback and takes air in the lobes where the hands are placed.

Accessory muscles in breathing—They are developed individually and in a group. Typically, sternocleidomastoid, scalene (anterior, middle, posterior) and also some other which helps in breathing are serratus anterior, pectorals, upper trapezius, latissimus dorsi, erector spine, quadratus lumborum, subclavius.

Combined costal and abdominal breathing:

- Deep and prolonged inspiration and expiration (active efforts)
- Balloon blowing exercises increases the strength and vital capacity of lungs
- Incentive spirometry is a small and handy instrument can be used for either inspiration or expiration strengthening exercises. Pursed lip breathing: Patient inhales through the nose with closed mouth, then forming a wide slit with lips (pursed lips), patient exhales slowly and smoothly for a greater period (ratio—inspiration: expiration 1:3). Because of the pursed lips, the air pressure from the mouth travel back in the spasmodic airways and alveoli and keep them open for a longer period allowing more removal of residual air.

Glossopharyngeal breathing (GPB-Frog like) was first observed in the late 1940s in polio patients at Rancho Los Amigo Hospital in Los Angeles, USA by Dr Clarence. This very useful technique is not very well known or practiced. As an analogy to positive pressure breathing used by amphibians, it is called frog breathing. The muscles of the mouth and pharynx are used to propel small volumes of air through the larynx into the lower lungs. The glottis is used to trap the air into the lungs while the next gulp of air being processed. The process is repeated, 8–10 times until a satisfactory breath is obtained. GPB can sustain ventilation for several hours in patients who are fully ventilator-dependent. "It is also useful for cough efficiency". It improves the voice and speech quality. Competitive free divers use this technique to increase lung volume and breathe holding time.

Paradoxical breathing (Reverse movement): Breathing movement in which the chest wall moves inside on inspiration and moves outside on expiration—reverse of the normal breathing movements. It is a life-threatening medical condition. The causes are multiple rib and sternum fractures, paralysis, chronic obstructive pulmonary disease (COPD), respiratory distress. The fractured fragments can pierce the pleura and lungs and can cause complications. Physiotherapy in paradoxical breathing—Pain relief including intercostal blocks, (avoid narcotics) followed by postural drainage with proper positioning and guarded slow and smooth breathing exercises to improve tidal volume and oxygenation. Patient needs ventilator.

Weaning from Ventilator

To achieve the ultimate goal of getting patient to breathe on their own, timing is critical. The sooner you liberate the patient from ventilator, the better but premature discontinuation can compromise gas exchange and lead to reintubation. One-third patients can not be weaned off on first attempt. Skillful judgment of physio is useful.

A gradual reduction of ventilator's support, starting with cutting back on supplemental oxygen support and eventually ending with extubation or tracheal decannulation was the tradition. Recently, a scientific-specific protocol approach developed by physiotherapists is well accepted. First ascertain how well the patient is healing from underlying disease. Patient is excited but ease the patient's fear of problems on weaning. Other factors to be resolved are pain, muscle fatigue, renal insufficiency and poor nutrition.

According to arterial blood gas (ABG) results, patient's pH should be 7.25 or greater. PaO_2 (partial pressure of arterial oxygen) should be 60 mm of Hg or greater. No more than 50% FiO_2 (fraction of inspired oxygen) and 8 cm H_2O. The PaO_2/FiO_2-P/F ratio an ideal predictor of oxygenation status and readiness to wean should be greater than 200. Additionally, the hemoglobin level should be at least 8 g/dL, magnesium, potassium and phosphorus should be within normal range.

Spontaneous breathing trial (SBT) is a test whereby patient attempts to breathe independently while still connected to ventilator. Trials are from 5–15 minutes, repeated 4 times a day.

"C" Circulation

Nervous system adjusts the diameter of our arteries. The blood pressure and the muscular contraction force, help blood to return from body parts to heart. After SCI, the arteries are wide open and blood pressure is lowered, muscle contraction-relaxation is hampered affecting blood circulation. These can produce the problems of i) Edema, ii) DVT-Deep Vein Thrombosis (blood clot in the vein usually in legs), iii) Pulmonary embolism (blood clot that has moved to lungs), iv) Orthostatic hypotension (blood pressure reduction in sitting-standing), v) Decreased heart rate vi) Reduced control of body temperature.

Physio can help improving circulation by Range of Motion (ROM) exercises of limbs and also by breathing exercises and thereby reducing the complications. At the end of the session the limbs are placed in "functional position".

17

Rehabilitative Medicine Services

Rehabilitation medicine includes:

- Restoration of physical and mental health
- Retraining for functional activities
- Prevention of disability
- Appliances for loss of functions
- Vocational retraining and placement
- Resettlement in the community.

In rehabilitation process, the concept of "Self-hope, self-help" and "nondependence" is on higher side than dependence on rehab services and welfare agencies.

From this part onwards, patient's active participation in the rehab process is the prime purpose along with the reception of rehab services for an altered self-sufficient satisfying life.

CUSTOMER CARE ASPECT

Mohandas Gandhi gave this life philosophy and "Customer is the most important…." Writings are found in some banks in India. As is with independence concept, the customer care is observed very well in USA and other countries. It is imperative and important to provide needed customer services to SCI patients.

ETHICS AND MEDICOLEGAL ISSUES

Ethics are based on morals and the values in life of a person. One should think that if we were SCI patient what sort of services and assistance we would expect from other persons. Keeping this in mind we should serve and help SCI patients in all aspects physically, mentally and financially.

Medicolegal issues are based on laws. Many countries including India have laws to protect the rights of the disabled persons. If the SCI patient do not get desired services, or if the treating professional made mistake due to ignorance, lack of skill or negligence, the patient has right to sue the hospital and the treating professional.

REHAB MEASURES FOR INDOOR PATIENTS

When the survival phase is almost over and the patient is entering in the settlement phase. The program is planned with the "Day cycle and Timing" concept. Everyone lives/leads life with a day cycle of 24 hours/day, with three phases.

18

Day Cycle Concept

INTRODUCTION

- Eight hours for self-care brushing, bathing, toilet, dressing, feeding, praying, social, sports
- Eight hours for earning or learning and housekeeping (here patient is learning how to get settled in the new lifestyle)
- Eight hours for sleep, rest, recreation and relaxation.

Because of the injury, the patient's day cycle is disturbed in particular and also of the family members, in general. During this settlement phase, patient, family, medical and rehab team, work hand in hand, harmony to rehabilitate the patient and set up a new day cycle and send the patient back to the home happily.

During "Day cycle", person/patient, interact with many persons, give and take help, care and share with each other. In this way, patient get adjusted with the available resources in that set up/situation within the family, society and at work. Patient should keep the list of needs ready. There are times when friends or family say, what help can we provide, patient immediately should ask for a help from the list, or request appropriate person for the help from the list.

Making a schedule for a particular day (e.g. program for February 24th) can help a patient/person to manage one's needs according to the time in the surroundings. Properly planned timing the lowers stress and is effective. Patient must start practicing from the beginning and from a good habit. Preferably an year's planner diary needs to be maintained. The need of searching and utilization of resources is preferably planned on previous eve (e.g. on 23rd February for 24th February).

DAY CYCLE WITH WHOLE DAY REHABILITATION PROGRAM

This type of program for SCI patients is unique and is one of the salient feature of Government Spine Institute. This planned program is executed from dawn to dusk. The students of UG/PG make the whole scene more energetic and enthuastic by taking part in actively in line program (Fig. 1).

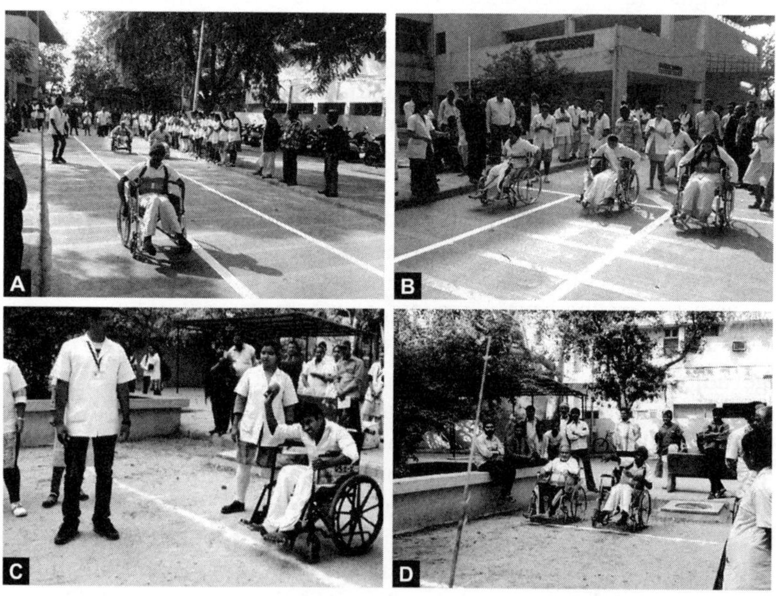

Fig. 1: Spinal cord injury patients playing sports: (A and B) Wheelchair racing; (C) Shot put; (D) Javelin throw

The whole day program at a glance:

Time	*Program*
6.00 am to 9.00 am	Getting ready. Self-care including brushing, bathing/sponging, toilet, dressing, meditation/prayers, breakfast
9.00 am to 10.30 am	Patient attends physiotherapy and occupational therapy department. Tilt table mobilization (Group therapy of sports and recreation for those who are on WC)
10.30 am to 12.30 pm	Patients on WC attend PT/OT department for muscle strengthening exercises. Balance, transfers and activity of daily living-training
12.30 pm to 2.00 pm	Back towards for lunch and resting
2.00 pm to 5.00 pm	Bedside PT/OT/ST/MSW and rehab services for bedridden patients. Periodical eval of patient and grand rehab round with professionals. Each patient is discussed for medical, social, vocational, rehab and necessary decisions are taken on the spot for further treatment
5.00 pm to 8.00 pm	Patients on WC are encouraged to sit in a garden-play and discuss their problems with other patients. TV programs in the wards and other entertainment programs
8.00 pm to 9.00 pm	Dinner in the wards. Then after a prayer/meditation and finally going to bed for a sleep

19

Cautious Care to Avoid Complications

Generally, complications occur after few months. Many complications hamper the progress and leads to morbidity, disability and death. Hence from the beginning, care is taken to avoid grave situations. It is reported that only 18.3% of patients did not experience secondary medical complications. The three most common complications that occur are pneumonia (34.3%), pressure sores (33.5%) and deep vein thrombosis (DVT 15%).

AUTONOMIC DYSREFLEXIA

Autonomic dysreflexia (AD) also known as autonomic hyperreflexia (T6 and above lesions) is a life-threatening situation and is a medical emergency. It is an automatic (involuntary) reaction to stimuli.

Common Causes

- Bladder distention
- Constipation with stool impaction
- Urinary tract infection (UTI)
- Noxious or painful stimuli—The stimuli are interrupted in their journey to the brain due to the transection of cord which results into a paradoxical stimulations of the autonomic nervous system
- Side effects of some certain psychoactive drugs can cause retention of urine and constipation.

Patient Exhibits

- High blood pressure

- Throbbing headache
- Nasal stuffiness
- Profuse sweating
- Flushing of skin above the lesion
- Facial erythema
- Blurred vision.

Steps to Stop Problems

- Sitting up patient with dangling leg position bed side
- Tight clothing and stockings be removed
- Relief from blocked catheter
- With anesthetic lubricant jelly, stool impaction be removed
- Sublingual nitrate or oral clonidine
- Ganglionic blockers to control sympathetic nervous system outflow
- Topical nitropaste is safe and is applied 1–2 inches on chest wall and is removed when BP is normal.

POSTURAL (ORTHOSTATIC) HYPOTENSION

When a patient assumes sudden sitting or standing position after a long lying position, patient's blood pressure suddenly falls—Systolic at least 20 mm Hg or diastolic 10 mm Hg of blood pressure. It is more likely in cervical and high thoracic lesions.

Patient exhibits dizziness, lightheadedness, giddiness, nausea, vomiting, headache, blurred vision, decrease in hearing, numbness, fainting.

Mechanism: Gravitational pooling of blood in the lower limbs results in reduced filling pressure at heart and lack of sympathetically mediated vasoconstriction.

Remedy: Immediately make the patient lie down, close eyes, and give patient to drink juice with salt and sugar. There should be slow progression to vertical position, i.e. elevation of the head off the bed. Gradual 5 degrees/day on tilt table mobilization, reclining wheel chair with elevating leg rest.

(In postural hypotension, patient is taken to lying from upright position whereas in autonomic dysreflexia, patient is made upright to reduce symptoms).

PRESSURE SORE-PRESSURE ULCER

Pressure sores are ulcerations of soft tissue caused by unrelieved pressure, friction and shearing forces. Pressure sores are subject to infection which can migrate to wound. Impaired sensation and inability to make positional changes are the two most influential factors in the development of pressure sores.

Management: Pressure sores are prevented with skin care: apply emollients to keep skin pliable, proper bed, proper positioning, weight relieving techniques. Sores/wounds are treated by dressing, debridement, whirlpool bath, skin grafts, ultraviolet radiation, infrared rays, laser scanner, ionization.

DEEP VEIN THROMBOSIS

Deep vein thrombosis (DVT) results from the development of a thrombus within deep vein. Blood clots in superficial veins called thrombophlebitis rarely cause serious problems. DVT often develop in calf and thigh vein. There is loss of pumping mechanism by lower limbs muscles. Prolonged immobilization (sleeping, sitting), smoking, age will increase the chances of occurrence.

The slow blood flow will allow higher concentration of pro-coagulants to develop in local area. Patient has local swelling, redness, part is hot and painful or tenderness on touch or squeeze. Prophylactic anticoagulant (heparin) plays important role. Other measures include turning, gentle passive range of motion exercises, elastic support stocking. Homan's sign (John Homans USA)—A positive sign is present when there is a pain in the calf muscle on forceful and abrupt dorsiflexion of patient's foot at ankle with knee flexed. A negative sign does not rule it out. The test is less used as it can potentially dislodge the thrombus and can cause problems. DVT diagnosis requires ultrasonic imaging and blood tests.

DVT is a life-threatening situation. The clot can break loose, travel through the blood stream to the lungs and block blood flow in the lungs (pulmonary embolism).

In an established case, the limb is rested in an elevated (above heart level) position and except active movements at other parts; exercises at the DVT area are avoided.

PNEUMONIA

Pneumonia is an inflammatory condition in the alveoli, caused by viruses and bacteria. It is due to decreased neuromuscular activities in the chest and abdomen. Those with tetraplegia may have decreased motor function in the diaphragm that impairs ventilation. Those with T5 and above level can have loss of intercostal and abdominals. Patients may have atelectasis (collapsed lungs with airlessness state) and aspiration (Aspiration pneumonia is a lung infection that develops after inhaling food, liquid or vomit in the lungs). It generally occurs after 5–7 years of injury.

The typical symptoms are cough, fever, chest pain, difficulty in breathing. It is diagnosed by X-ray and sputum culture. Patients are treated by antibiotics and rest.

Preventive measures include PFT check-up every year, influenza vaccination and patient should perform different types of "Breathing exercises" religiously daily.

ASPIRATION

Food, fluid, secretions entering in the respiratory system from the trachea. It may lead to pneumonia and death, depending upon the volume, particle size, composition and underline patient's health status (hospitalization, depressed, semiconsciousness and impaired gag reflex (laryngeal spasm preventing choking). Eat or drink with consciousness to avoid food/fluid entering into the trachea.

DEPRESSION

Depression is a mood disorder. Mood is an emotional feeling. Moods affect our behavior and our attitude towards life. Patient feels hopeless, worthless and guilty. Depression may be short- or long-term. It may be sudden or slow. Other people see changes before the patient sees it. Patient's problems are:

- Sadness and grieve for the way the life was before
- Become angry and blame themselves or others
- Have hard time adjusting to being dependent
- Not be able to do desired things on their own

- Lose interest in doing things
- Lose or increase appetite and lose or increase weight
- Cannot sleep soundly
- Feel tired and sleepy during day hours
- Be restless, irritable, withdrawn
- Concentration, memory, decision making is affected.

Management of Depression

Medication: Antidepressant are started and stopped as per the advice of a psychiatrist.

Psychotherapy: Psychological counseling should be done individually or in a group. All rehab professionals will give counseling-motivation before the treatment. Talk to patient, family and care givers about the realistic goal and how to cope up to gain it.

Patient's brain should not be kept idle (An idle mind is devil's workshop). It should be involved inactive participation for talking and walking (moving), group gathering, socializing, curative, creative and vocational activities.

Contracture

Soft tissues (muscles, ligaments, capsules) have an elastic property of lengthening and shortening on movement. Body parts with spasm, spasticity, inability and if they are not moved, they lose elasticity and following problems occur:

Tightness: The tissues are tight but can be passively lengthened to its full length.

Contractures: Tissues cannot be lengthened passively (tissues are converted into nonelastic fibrous tissues). Contractures need surgical release.

Deformity: The body is not in an alignment and is deformed. As the body is kept in a position of ease, patients develop deformity in hip-knee flexion, leg in adduction, internal rotation and foot in equines. Shoulder-elbow in flexion, arm in internal rotation.

Disability: The deformed body creates further disability. It will be more difficult for patient and the caretaker to move/lift body for transfers and activities of daily living.

Daily, active-passive range of motion exercises, body movement, positioning and splinting will prevent these problems.

PAIN AND DYSESTHESIA

'Dys' means not normal, 'Aesthesis' means sensation-abnormal sensation. Patient has below the lesion, sensation of burning (acid under the skin), itching, electric shock, pins and needle, sharp-stabbing-shooting pain which may follow dermatomal pattern, most common in cauda equina injury.

It is managed conservatively with drugs and transcutaneous electric nerve stimulation (TENS). Severe cases needs severing nerve roots, posterior rhizotomy.

URINARY TRACT INFECTION

Urinary tract infection (UTI) is a common problem with SCI patients more with female patients. Common causes are continuous catheterization, nonaseptic catheter insertion, incomplete voiding. In females, urethra is nearer to anus and is shorter, hence *E. Coli* easily enters urethra. Patient has fever, chills and painful urination.

After urine culture, necessary antibiotics are given. Genital area is kept cleaned. Intake of adequate fluid to flush the bladder and urethra.

RENAL CALCULI (KIDNEY STONE)

Stagnant urine form crystals of mineral mass (oxalate, calcium, phosphorus) that combine to form stone. It is more common in male, in patient with complete lesions and in patients using indwelling catheter.

Patient has lower abdominal pain, back pain, painful urination, blood in urine, nausea (vomiting), fatigue, fever, loss of appetite. It is diagnosed with KUB X-ray.

Small stones can be flushed out with urine by plenty of water drinking, by saline drip. Big stones are removed with lithotripsy (High energy shock waves that break stone into stone dust) and with surgery. Drink more water, lemon-orange juice. Avoid eating meat, eggs, fish, spinach, nuts and wheat bran. Complete voiding by manual pressure on lower abdomen to prevent residual urine in bladder.

HETEROTOPIC OSSIFICATION

Heterotopic ossification (HO) is extra-articular, extracapsular calcium deposition in the soft tissues adjacent to large joints, e.g. hip, knee. It is caused by tissue hypoxia secondary to circulatory stasis, overstretching, aggressive massage, local pressure and microtrauma. Affected part is painful, swollen and hot with restriction in motion. Entrapped nerve (femoral, ulnar) or vein will have their symptoms.

Diagnosis is confirmed with X-ray. In an established case, rest is recommended. After the resolution of symptoms, careful gentle exercises are started. PT/OT will find out a customized position for sitting. Surgical resection has chances of reoccurrence.

OSTEOPOROSIS AND FRACTURES

Patient lose bone density, bones are porous, brittle and are likely to break. Osteopenia is an intermediate condition. It is diagnosed by Dual-energy X-ray Absorptiometry (DXA) scanning. About 80% of SCI have osteoporosis. Most of the loss is in the trabecular bones (femur, tibia).

Causes are lack of loading, inhibits bone building cells, lack of movement, sluggish blood flow, less consumption of balanced food, hormonal alteration.

Treatment: Calcium citrate, vitamin D3, Sun rays, exercises and weight bearing—loading on bones (both are done with a great care to avoid fracture), functional electrical stimulation, low intensity vibration, healthy diet.

SPASTICITY

After spinal cord injury, the nerve cells (connected to muscle) become disconnected from brain and normal reflexes become exaggerated on stimuli. The bladder, kidney infection and skin breakdown will increase the problem.

Spasticity can be controlled with daily gentle passive range of motion exercises, ice application, strengthening exercises of opposite group, surgery-partial rupturing of respective nerve, partial release of spastic muscle tendon-tenotomy, rhizotomy.

CARDIOVASCULAR DISEASE

SCI persons generally live sedentary lifestyle and are at higher risk. Upper extremity exercises (Pull ups and Push ups), breathing exercises pranayama, meditation and mobility will help reduce the problems of patients.

HYPER-/HYPO-THERMIA

Because of the altered function of the autonomic nervous system, the body temperature fluctuates according to the surrounding temperature. If the patient is in a hot room, person will have hyperthermia and in a cold room, patient will have hypothermia. Higher lesions have more problems. Treat the person to reduce the problem and provide opposite hot or cold surrounding atmosphere.

20

Morbidity and Mortality

Preventable complications lead to morbidity and mortality and vice a versa.

Morbidity: Abnormally gloomy (depressingly darkness with dejection feeling) or unhealthy state of mind with inactivity.

Morbidity in spinal cord injury (SCI) is due to pain, spasticity, pressure sores, postural hypotension, fractures and respiratory complications. The higher incidence of morbidity is influenced by low educational level, low income, lack of awareness regarding complications, lack of follow-up, lack of motivation, lack of vocational engagement, lack of sociocultural involvement, lack of predischarge home visit, lack of specialized centers, poor community setup with poor infrastructure and patient spending more time in bed.

Mortality: Before World War II, most SCI died within weeks due to pressure sores, urinary dysfunction, and respiratory infection. The advent of modern antibiotics, plastics, latex, surgical procedures and the type of rehabilitation measures, are the greatest indicator of long-term survival.

Overall 85% of SCI who survive the first 24 hours are alive 10 years later (In developed countries with better financial favors and facilities for care). The first leading cause of death is pneumonia. Second cause is nonischemic heart disease. Third is due to external causes-unintentional injury, suicide and homicide.

The morbidity and mortality rate is higher in patients with low education, low economy, nonemployment and in underdeveloped countries with poor infrastructure facility for indoor and outdoor mobility and accessibility. Because of that patient is compelled to remain confined to bed.

(A paper presented in IAP Conference by Nalina Gupta, John Solomon, Kavita Raja).

21

Clinical Psychological Counseling Services

A psychiatrist treats patients mainly with Medicines and holds MD degree in Psychiatry.

Clinical psychologist treats patients with counseling and holds masters degree in clinical psychology (Learning program is at BM Institute Ashram road, Ahmedabad and De-addiction center, Bhat-Indira Bridge, Ahmedabad).

Spinal cord injury (SCI) patients have feeling of dejection and depression which comes in their way of treatment. To instill the feeling that they can be still useful member is important.

SCI is such a devastating condition that it not only damages the body functioning but also destroys patient's social status, financial foundation and the self-esteem, producing a grave situation with a dark future ahead, giving a setback in person's psychology with a depression. Patient needs careful handling to come out of it and to cope up with the situation for the rehab process.

Sadness is a blue feeling that there is some major problem with personal loss which should not be confused with depression.

Patient undergoes these stages:

- *Denial/Disbelief:* Refuses to accept the loss and may see the injury as an illness similar to a cold or flu with fever that will soon pass away with time.
- *Anger:* Feelings of displeasure and may lash out verbally or may become physically violent. Patient may become angry to himself, to others, even to the God.
- *Bargaining:* Acceptance may come with the belief that he will be rewarded for the prayers and the hard work in therapy and will eventually recover.

- *Depression:* Patient has extreme sadness, inactivity, problems with concentration and cognition, appetite and sleep disorders, feelings of dejections-worthlessness. Person becomes introverts with "Self-talk", My life is over, No one will accept-love or respect me, everyone will take advantage of me as I can't defend. These unrealistic Self talk leads to severe depression and does not allow for disability acceptance. Patient may have suicidal thoughts.
- *Acceptance:* Earlier the better. Grieving usually ends and he start accepting a reality of the current condition and to find out a meaning in life as a SCI person. Acceptance is the turning point from where "Real Reshaping" starts.

Adjustment requires understanding of the self with the surroundings, finding out the resources and to modify it as per personal need. Adjustments are needed at every front—personal, family, social and vocational.

COUNSELING

Because humans are capable of cognition and comprehension, the rehab team should explain in suitable terms, the relevant details of the injury, damage, pathology, prognosis, biomechanics, goal settings in order to harness greater cooperation and higher motivation from patient (Hill DA). Rehab professionals's role is unique, on one hand, it resembles to a Medical scientist and on the other hand to an Educational psychologist (Dr Mokashi MG).

Counseling is the foundation of reshaping and resettlement. In a group with all the Rehab professionals (Rehab round), patient's problems are discussed and plans are planned to do counseling. One and all, including relatives will do counselling prior and during their treatment. Person's mind is the driving force for all the activities. Convincing the patient for problems and to activate to put efforts with solutions is the counseling. Patient initially needs "Sympathy" (sharing the feelings in sorrow) to soothe emotions but afterward they need "Empathy" (not only sharing feelings but also to discuss the problems, to care, guide and assist constantly till the person becomes happier again).

In the early phase, patient has a hope to go back to previous state. This Hope is harnessed for the efforts for exercises. Approximately after 3–4 months, patient may not show recovery in the muscle strength, at this stage, patients' efforts needs to be diverted for the reshaping and rehabilitation with the available potentials. After 3–4 months "Don't wait for cure, care to get settled with what is available".

FAMILY ADJUSTMENT

Although family members have not lost their ability to walk or do hand work like patient; they also grieve and face stress with anxiety. They will have a loss in the way their life was before. They will have to do workout for family finances, house-kitchen modifications for accessibility, and adaptations for cooking, change the work schedule or quit the job. They will have to help the patient for personal needs including lifting, help in transfers, help for bladder and bowel, food and fluid.

FAMILY SUPPORT

When patient gets back home, the relatives have an all powerful position and can make or break the patient's progress. They need to understand the problems faced by the victim of SCI to help him in a best way. If they smother with overhelp (e.g. propelling WC and not allowing patient to propel, they may make him handicap and if they offer too little help, life may become too difficult and patient may give up trying.

22

Patient's Partner or Caregiver's Services

Majority of spinal cord injury (SCI) patients need lifelong assistance for their daily activities. This ranges from bathing-dressing, toilet-bladder-bowel, lifting-transporting, food and fluid services. Unlike hospice (terminally ill) patients, these patients need physical and emotional assistance for a very long period of time. For all these services, a caregiver is needed round the clock. They may be life partner, family member or paid attendant. In the poor and middle class families, these services are provided by family member whereas rich family affords to hire a paid attendant. It is observed that for male patient the spouse assists and for female patient paid attendant is hired. It is recommended to find out a suitable caregiver, right from the beginning of the rehab program in the hospital and they need to be trained how to get involved in the rehab process.

These caretakers are educated about the body functioning, spinal cord injury and the complications of the SCI. They are also informed about how and how much assistance to be given, how to encourage patient to do the possible tasks independently. Since these services to the patient is for a long time, they are trained how to lift and transfer the patient with minimal energy expenditure and to avoid the stress, strain and injury to their body with the biomechanical principles. During lifting and transferring the patient, they must tighten the tummy and keep the patient nearer to their body to avoid injury to the back.

CARING THE CAREGIVER

As the assistance is needed for a long time, caregiver also faces many physical and psychological problems. To avoid such problems, they must do the following:

- Take nutritive balanced foods and fluids to remain healthy and happy
- Find out time to rest and relax from a tiring physical/psychological task
- Revive and rejuvenate brain with recreational programs
- Do fitness exercises to remain strong and sustainable
- Do pranayama and meditation to maintain cool and calm brain
- Find out alternative adjustment for sexual issues.

23

Student's Support Services

Students who are in their teenage are full of energy and enthusiasm. When students are with the patients, they transfer this vigor to the patient and provide a fighting force. At Government Spine Institute, Government Prosthetic and Orthotic College, students are helping hands to the professionals who are serving patients. It is observed that, if guided well, learners are good servers. Being an academic and research center, students take up dissertation for their PG studies and staff carry out research projects to improve rehabilitation services to care patients.

24

Physiotherapy Services

Physiotherapist (PT) is a medical profession, concerned with the remedy of impairment, disability, handicap and promotion of mobility-movement, functional ability and quality of life through examination, evaluation, diagnosis, interpretation and intervention using physical agents—heat, cold, water, electricity for therapy and electrodiagnosis, sun rays, counseling, soft tissue mobilization-manipulations, therapeutic exercises and selective use of medicines.

According to Gujarat State Council for Physiotherapy— "Physiotherapy" means a branch of modern medical science which includes examination, assessment, interpretation, physical diagnosis, planning and execution of treatment and advice to any person for the purpose of preventing, correcting, alleviating and limiting dysfunction, acute and chronic bodily malfunction, including life-saving measures via chest physiotherapy in the intensive care units, curing physical disorders or disability, promoting physical fitness, facilitating healing and pain relief and treatment of physical and psychosomatic disorder through modulating physiological and physical response using exercises, physical agents, activities and devices including mobilization, manipulations, mechanical, electrical, and thermal agents, including therapeutic ultrasound and therapeutic LASER, and electrotherapy including electrophysiology for diagnosis, treatment and prevention." (*Ref. https://gujhealth.gujarat.gov.in/images/pdf/Act/gujarat-act-no18-2011-physiotharapy.pdf*)

According to Delhi Council for Physiotherapy and Occupational therapy Bill 1997—"Physiotherapy" means physiotherapeutic system of medicine which includes examination, treatment, advice and instructions to any person preparatory to or for the purpose of or in connection with movement dysfunction, bodily malfunction, physical disorder, disability, healing and pain from trauma and disease, physical and mental conditions using physical agents including exercise, mobilization, manipulations, mechanical and electrotherapy, activity and devices or diagnosis, treatment and prevention. (*Ref. http://delhiassembly.nic.in/aspfile/bills passed/141997.htm*)

According to Maharashtra State OTPT council—"Physiotherapy" means a branch of modern medical science which includes examination, assessment, interpretation, physical diagnosis, planning and execution of treatment and advice to any person for the purpose of preventing, correcting, alleviating and limiting dysfunction, acute and chronic bodily malfunction including life-saving measures via chest physiotherapy in the intensive care unit, curing physical disorders or disability, promoting physical fitness, facilitating healing and pain relief and treatment of physical and psychosomatic disorders through modulating physiological or physical response using physical agents, activities and devices including exercise, mobilization, manipulation, therapeutic ultrasound, electric and thermal agents and electrotherapy for diagnosis, treatment and prevention. (*Ref. http://www.msotptcouncil.com/OTPTAct.aspx*)

Though all members have role to play at every stage of rehab process, Physio's have active role in both survival and settlement sections of rehab team.

25

Physiotherapy in the Ward

EVALUATION

Patient is evaluated for the potential and problems.

Subjective

History is taken with complete information about the injury and the problems from the patient.

Objective

Objective assessment of muscle strength gradation (0 to 5) in lower motor lesions, in upper motor lesions voluntary control at joints is assessed. Spasticity is graded with Modified Ashworth scale. Myotomes, dermatomes and reflexes are assessed. Bladder-bowel status is obtained; range of motion (ROM) at joints, contractures-tightness-deformity (CTD) is measured. Skin is inspected for breakage and bedsore. Balance status, transfer activities achieved.

Assessment

Assessment and analysis of the data to find out the level of ability and disability and thereby deciding the neurological level.

Finally, patient is placed on the ASIA scale.

Plan

Planning for short- and long-term goals.

EDUCATION

Patient, relatives, caretakers are educated about the problem, body-brain functioning, goals and how to cope up to put efforts in right direction, care to prevent the complications.

TREATMENT

Therapeutic exercises are planned scientifically, as per the patient's ability and disability, with the recovery, treatment plans are modified.

- *Exercises:* Passive, assisted-active-resisted range of motion exercises are given
- *Breathing:* Diaphragmatic, costal, localized and accessory muscles exercises with huffing and coughing techniques are taught
- *Upper limbs:* For paraplegics, upper limbs will take over the work of lower limbs for ambulations, transfers, wheel chair mobility, hence they are hypertrophied
- *Log rolling:* Patient, caretakers are trained for log rolling of body every 2 hours
- *Functional positioning:* How to place the body parts in functional positions
- Skin inspection with a mirror with long handle.

Bladder and bowel training

Education

- Knowledge is given to know about the type (upper motor or lower motor)
- Intake—Fluid to flush the bladder and fiber food for motion movement
- Timings—Avoid drinking more fluid in late evening to avoid urination in night
- Amount—More fluid in summer due to perspiration. Less in winter
- Skill- training

Bladder

- Habit formation of voiding at regular intervals (2 hourly) to avoid accidents
- Self-catheterization technique
- Placing hot water bag on lower abdomen before urination
- Pulling pubic hair to initiate urination
- Pressing portion of lower abdomen (supra-pubic Crede's maneuver) or abdominal straining (Valsalva maneuver) during urination to empty bladder completely.

Bowel

- Habit formation of bowel, preferably daily in the morning
- Use of laxative/suppository placing, if there is constipation
- Stool removable with gloved fingers, if there is impaction.

26

Physiotherapy in the Department

Patients as per their medical-surgical status will be taken to the PT/ OT department.

Operated cases—Patient is made to sit within 3 days as per tolerance.

Patients with stable fractures (nonoperated) and stable medical conditions are taken on stretcher for tilt table mobilization after 3–4 weeks.

Patients with cervical tractions are taken on stretcher for tilt table mobilization after 6 weeks with a cervical orthosis, upon removal of traction.

PROGRAMS IN PHYSIOTHERAPY DEPARTMENT

Therapeutic exercises are not body building gym exercises but are "Scientifically" designed after evaluating patient's problems and the potentials.

Gradual-graded Tilt Table Mobilization (Fig. 1)

After 3–4 weeks of injury, patient with stable vertebral fracture is taken on tilt table from a stretcher and the table is tilted to 5 degrees. Patient will be on the table for 15 minutes and the tilting is increased by 5 degrees everyday. From 50 degrees onwards till 90 degrees, patient will attend OT department.

During tilted position, if patient has symptoms of postural hypotension (nausea, vomiting, sweating, giddiness due to "postural hypotension") patient is lowered down to horizontal position, eyes are closed, good ventilation is given and fluid with sugar/salt is provided.

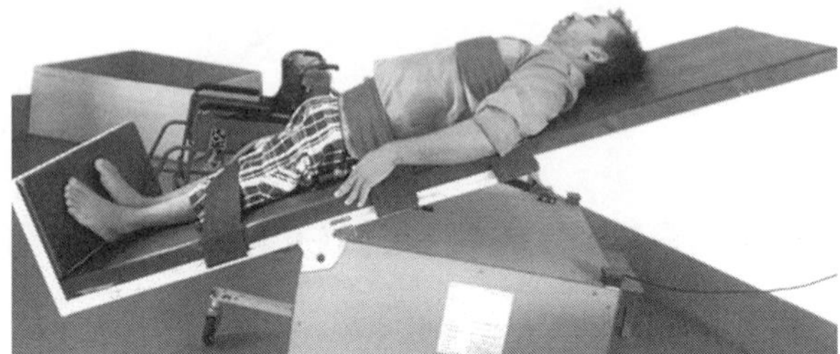

Fig. 1: Gradual-graded tilt table mobilization
(*Source:* Dr Dilip Patel, Dr SL Rai and Dr SP Mehta presented a scientific paper on "Effects of gradual early tilt table mobilization in Dorsal and lumbar stable fractures with cord involvement" in the National Physiotherapy Conference held at Kolkata in1983).

Pull Ups

Pull ups are done by pulling the body up with a handle attached to a chain above in the ceiling. The exercises are done with patients sitting in WC in a group of 8–10 patients. Along with the upper limbs strengthening, patient enjoys group interactions and the competitive moods (Fig. 2).

Push Ups

Push up is done with push up blocks or pushing body up on arm rest of the WC. Push ups in a group, will strengthen the upper limbs with group interactions benefits.

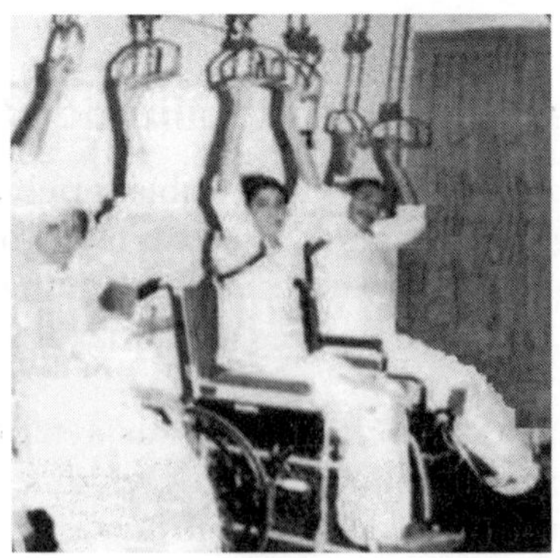

Fig. 2: Upper limb exercises "pull ups"

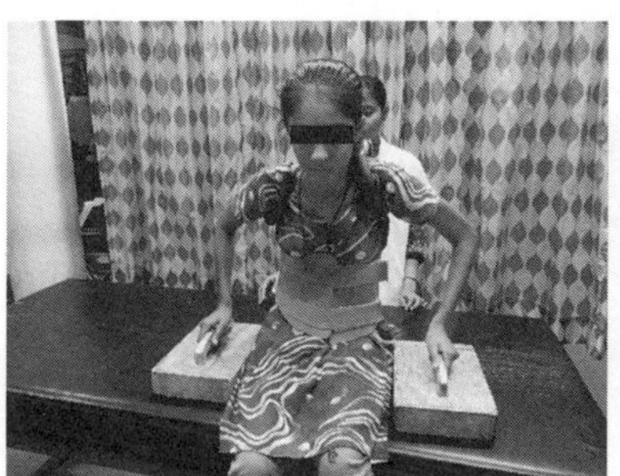

Fig. 3: Active push-ups using push-up blocks

Suspension Exercises

Suspension frame exercises for specific muscles (quadratus lumborum, lattisimus dorsi) or muscles with 2 grade power.

Specific Muscles Strengthening

Quadratus lumborum: Active then resistive work with pulling unilateral pelvis alternatively in lying and in standing; it is useful to pull one leg up (hip hiking) and clear the ground during walking with walker or cane.

Latissimus dorsi: Active and resistive work of shoulder extension, adduction, internal rotation. It is useful for "Shuffle gait" with crutches.

Shoulder adductors, elbow extensors, grip muscles strengthening, needed for crutch/frame walking, transfers and wheel chair maneuvering.

Balance Training (Fig. 4)

Training with tipping and supporting trunk and body will gain the sitting and standing balance. Trunk balance is useful to free upper limbs to do activities of daily living.

Muscle Strengthening Techniques

Isometric muscle work (*Iso* means same, *Metric* means length): Muscle contraction with no change in muscle length and no movement at joint.

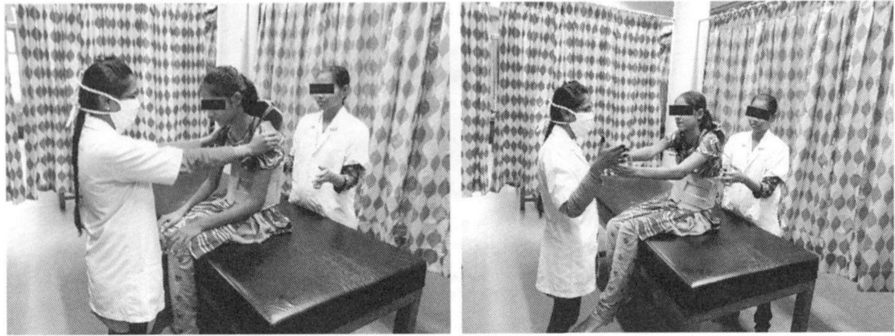

Fig. 4: Balance training and active reach-out exercises

Static muscle work is a pure active contraction without movement at joint but there is no resistance to the contracting muscle, e.g. Patient sitting in a long sitting position and contracting quadriceps actively (Quadricep's active work).

Isometric muscle work is a strong muscle contraction against resistance (gravity or weight) without movement at joint, e.g. Patient sitting at the edge of a table and holding knee straight with 2 kg weight (Quadricep's resistive holding work).

(Static is an active contraction; Isometric is contraction against resistance with maximal effort).

Isotonic muscle work (*Iso* means same, *Tonic* means tone)*:* Muscle contraction with lengthening or shortening of length and with movements at joint.

Eccentric muscle work: Muscle is contracting but simultaneously muscle is lengthening, i.e. the origin and insertion are going away from each other. For example, patient is sitting on the edge of a table—lowering the leg "gradually" with 2 kg weight from straight knee. Movement is slow and controlled and not dropping suddenly (Eccentric work of Quadriceps). Since the energy consumption is less in eccentric work than concentric work and person needs more concentration and consciousness, this form of exercise is useful in the rehabilitating muscles and in sport injury.

Concentric muscle work: Muscle is contracting and muscle is shortening, i.e. the origin and insertion are coming closer. For example, patient is sitting on the edge of a table—taking the lowered leg with 2 kg weight to knee straight position (Concentric work of Quadriceps).

Isokinetic Exercises: Iso means same, *kinesis* means motion (speed). A machine designed with high technology, where the speed of moving part of the machine remains same offering variables resistance to the

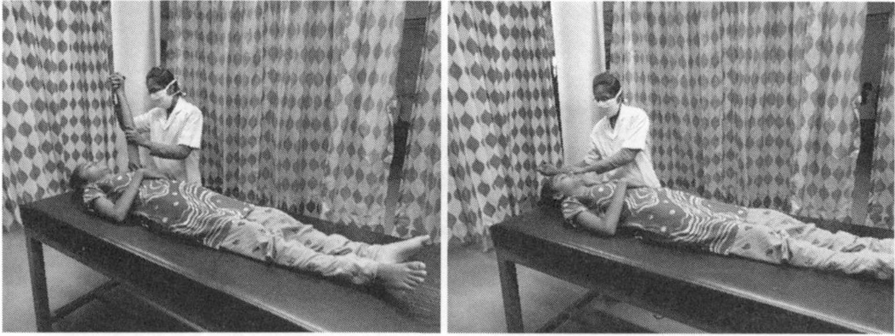

Fig. 5: Upper extremity exercises

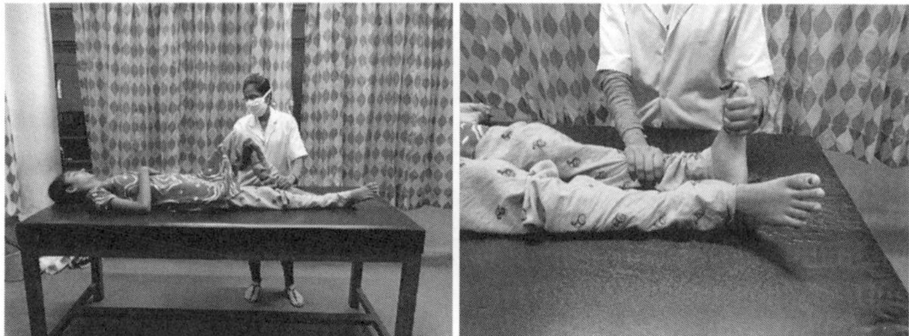

Fig. 6: Lower extremity exercises

working muscles as much the resistance a muscle can take up at that angle of a moving joint.

Stretching

Tight soft tissues are gently stretched passively. Some muscles can also be stretched with body weight position, e.g. Hip flexors in prone position.

Important: Tenodesis—With C6 lesion, there is an active wrist extension but no wrist and finger flexion, in this situation, it is wise to allow finger flexors to get tightness-contractures or don't stretch out, if it is there, this will produce "Tenodesis action" (On active wrist extension, patient will have functional grip with tight finger flexors). Tenodesis splint keeps wrist in extension, with flexed fingers, patient will have functional grip." Blessings in disguise."

Mat Exercises

To initiate and improve balance and transfer activities MAT exercises plays major role. Examples of mat exercises are shown in Figures 7 and 8.

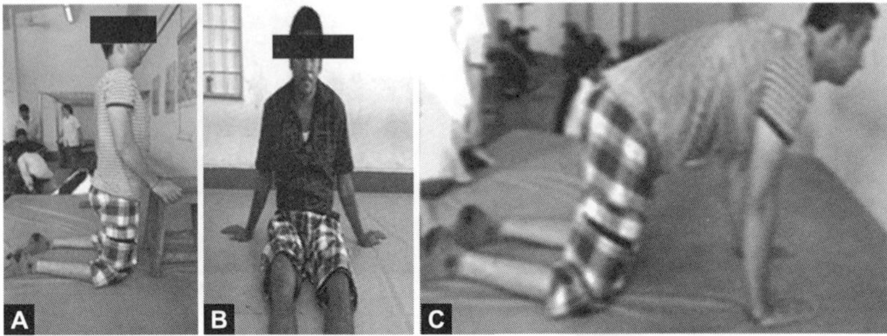

Fig. 7A to C: MAT exercises: (A) Kneeling; (B) Long sitting; (C) Prone kneeling

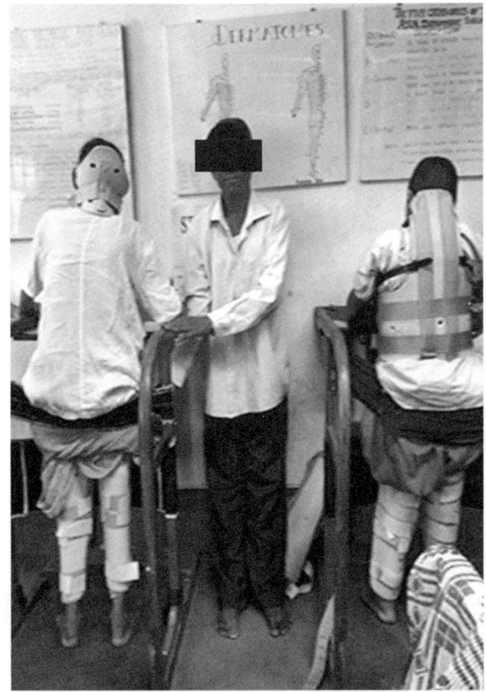

Fig 8: Quadruplegic (left) and paraplegic (right) patients practicing standing in standing frame

Breathing

Generalized, localized and exercises for accessory muscles (Fig. 9).

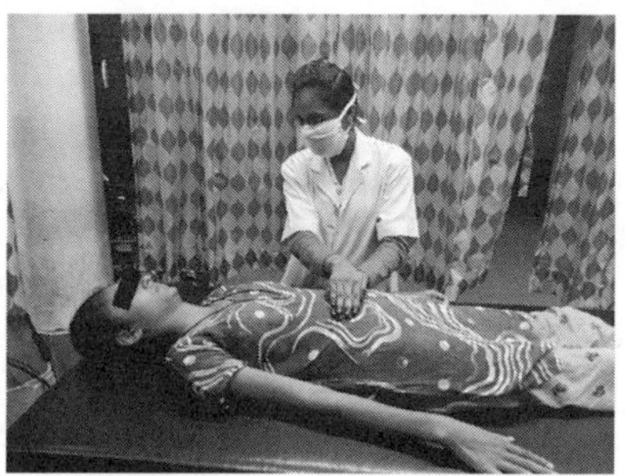

Fig. 5: Diaphragmatic breathing

GAIT TRAINING (GT)

Human locomotion is termed as a "Gait" in medical terminology. From a quadripedal (walking like animals), we have evolved to bipedal walking (walking on two legs—Upper limbs have no obligation for mobility and are free for activity for daily living and other creative works). Every individual has unique Gait pattern with the habit formation. Gait evaluation provides information to physiotherapist about the person's muscular weakness, soft tissue tightness, short limb, pain, paralysis, or diseases which help therapist to plan the program of gait training.

Normal Gait Cycle

Stance phase (60%): It is the time during which the foot is on the ground. Normal gait requires stability in stance phase, a means of progression and energy conservation. During progression, potential energy is converted into kinetic energy.

- Contact—Heel strike, knee is extended and ankle is in neutral position
- Initial stance—15 degrees of knee flexion, 15 degrees of plantar flexion. Hamstrings and dorsiflexors control the movement. Quadriceps and gluteal muscles maintain stability
- Mid stance—Full weight bearing, knee is extended and ankle is neutral. Triceps surae controls the tibial advancement
- Terminal stance—Heel off. Knee flexes 35 degrees, ankle plantar flexes to 20 degrees
- Preswing—Toes off.

Double support: When both feet are on ground (10% inclusive of 60% stance) (With the increase in speed of walking/running, double stance reduces).

Swing phase (40%): It is the time during which the foot is off the ground. Much of the kinetic energy for the swing phase is provided by inertia, which is assisted and augmented by plantarflexors (85%) and hip flexors (15%).

- Acceleration to mid swing—Quadriceps contraction prevents heel from rising too high and helps to initiate forward swing of the leg
- Mid swing to deceleration—Hamstrings and anterior cruciate ligament control the speed for heel strike (In anterior cruciate injury, emphasis is given to hamstrings strengthening for this reason).

In a gait cycle, during push off, the whole body rises up and then lowers down. When our right leg is going forward, the left arm also goes forward; hence there is alternate upper trunk rotation during gait.

Gait Analysis/Gait Laboratory

Gait can be analyzed with:

- Naked eye observation of person's gait from front, back and from side
- Still photography of different phases of gait cycle
- Videography of different phases of gait cycle (slow motion study)
- High-tech electronic gait analyzer with EMG facility.

Gait analyzer is equipped with many cameras for gait recording. The mat on which the person is walking is with pressure sensitive sensors which detect the amount of pressure a person is putting during walking. The invisible pressure is made visible on computer screen. Time interval is also detected of the swing and stance phase. This analyzer is also having facility of an attached EMG machine which detects the amount of recruitment of different muscles during different phases of the gait. In this technology era, every aspect of the gait is mapped, measured and minutely analyzed on computer.

Gait Trainer (Fig. 10)

The patient's trunk is harnessed with a belt and then hanged above on the machine. The length of the hanging rope can be increased or decreased as per the tolerance of the patient for weight bearing.

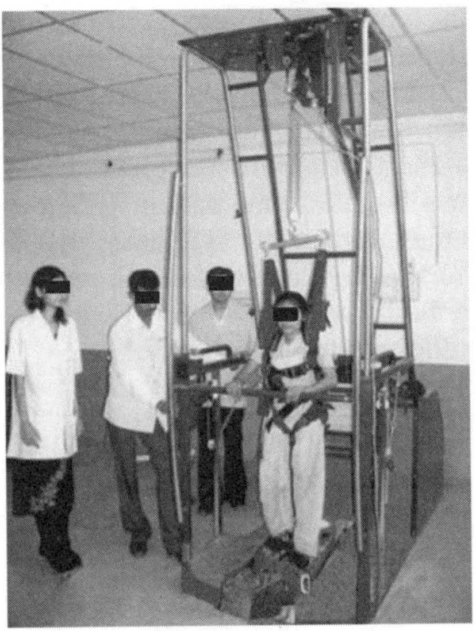

Fig. 10: Gait trainer

The feet are placed on the feet boards which moves mechanically, alternatively like a leg movement during walking. There is also a facility of an attached muscle stimulator which stimulates the weak muscles during walking. The practice on this machine not only facilitates weight bearing but the rhythmical motion of legs is also gained.

Abnormal Gaits

- Antalgic (limping) Gait: Patient leans on the painful side. Stance phase is reduced
- Waddling Gait: Pelvis drops on opposite side of the leg on stance. Hip abductor of the stance phase can't hold the pelvis from dropping
- High steppage Gait: Patient lifts the leg higher in foot drop to clear the ground
- Equinus Gait: Affected leg is apparently longer due to fixed equinus deformity of the foot with gastrosoleus contracture. Body rises up during stance phase
- Calcaneus Gait: There is no push off due to weakness of gastrocnemius soleus
- Hand to knee Gait: Patient locks the knee with hand in quadriceps weakness
- Gluteal (backward) lurch: In gluteus maximus weakness, the hip goes back in stance of the affected leg. In hip abductor weakness, it is waddling
- Intermittent claudication Gait: Patient can walk some distance and needs rest to walk again. Patient can't walk fast or far
- Neurogenic claudication is observed in spinal stenosis. Vascular claudication is due to arterial insufficiency in muscles (Atherosclerosis).

SCI patients are first given pregait training exercises and as per the assessment findings, the GT program is progressed.

As per the muscle strength, different orthosis are given:

- HKAFO (hip, knee, ankle, foot orthosis) in whole limb weakness
- KAFO (knee, ankle, foot orthosis) (Scott-Greig orthosis). With KAFO, patient is trained to stand with hips in hyperextension
- AFO (ankle, foot orthosis) with weakness of foot and ankle

After proper assessment, some patients are given posterior knee guard (PKG) and toe raising splint (TRS) (Fig. 9). GT in a gait trainer.

- Patient is harnessed and hanged from above with weight bearing on feet as tolerated.
- Parallel bar standing with or without orthosis.
- GT in parallel bars (Fig. 10).
- GT with a walker (frame).
- GT with two sticks (canes) to with one stick to independent walking. Human help is gradually withdrawn to make patient independent.

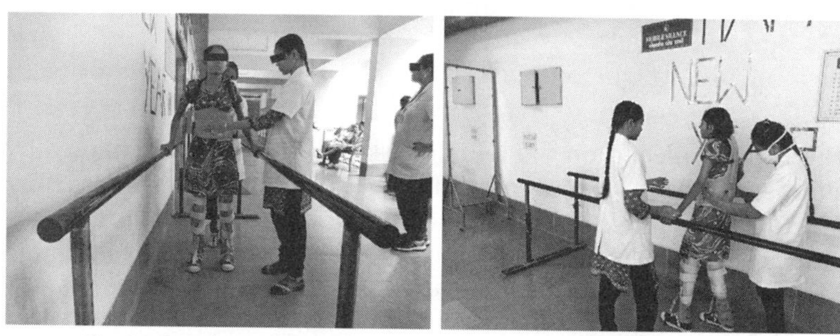

Fig. 11: Standing and walking in parallel bars assisted by physiotherapists

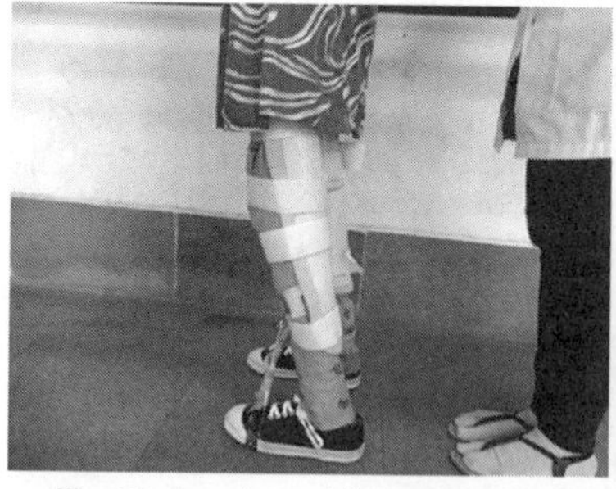
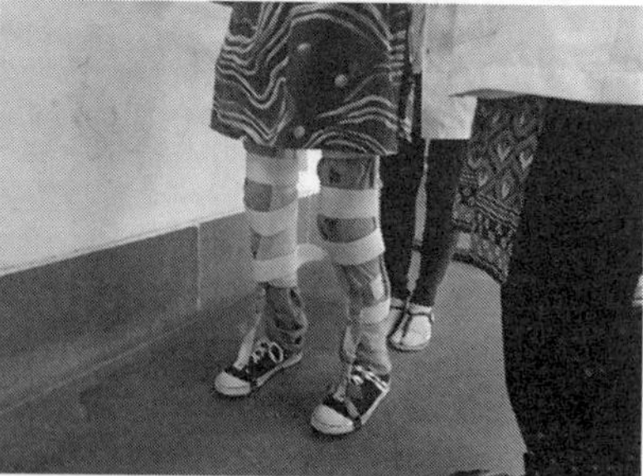

Fig. 12: A patient with posterior knee guard (PKG) and toe raising splint (TRS) being assisted for gait training by physiotherapists

27

Allied Sciences/Alternative (Complementary) Medicine

It has been observed that in India and in many countries, patients with chronic medical ailment go from one to another medical discipline for getting relief. It is essential that Physio-Rehab professionals know some basics of these disciplines.

Alternative medicines: Yoga, Ayurveda, Naturopathy, Acupressure, Acupuncture, Magnetotherapy. They claim to have healing and health effects on body without using modern medicine.

YOGA (ASANA-PRANAYAMA-MEDITATION): A SCIENTIFIC EXPLANATION

Yoga—(1) Yug means to join, a Harmony of body-mind-soul (union with Divine), (2) The stilling of the changing states of mind (chitta-vrutti nirodh), (3) Expertise in work is yoga (karmeshu kaushalam is yoga). Maharishi Patanjali (neither a doctor nor a scientist) derived and designed yoga in ancient time. Present science accepts it as a sound skill for health and happiness.

Medical, Surgical and Rehab measures, objectively obtains recovery, rehabilitation and Yoga, Pranayama, Meditation supports the process and sustains lifelong physical-psychological-emotional equilibrium.

Aerobics strengthens systems of body.

Yoga synchronizes systems of body. Harmony of body and brain. Synthesis of self with savior; Connects consciousness with cognition.

Our body organs work with different systems and speeds, e.g. brain thinking, respiration, heart beating, sight, hearing. Yoga helps to regulate rhythm in systems. Yoga is not only useful for patient, but it is also needed for patient's partner and caregiver as they have to remain mentally sharp and sound and physically strong.

Spine is considered to be the important body organ in Yoga as well. The seven chakras meaning wheel or turning but in yoga the meaning is Vortex or whirlpool. These seven chakras are energy points in the subtle body (not physical body). They are located at the physical counter parts of the major plexuses of arteries, veins, nerves, glands. The three Nadis Ida, Pingala, Shushumna pass through them from down to upwards with the life force (Prana) or vital energy. When chakras and spine are in alignment, the energy force flows well.

The "Ashtangyog" ladder of "Sage Patanjali" for psychosomatic ailment-Prevention and Elimination for "Wellbeing"

Stage-8: Samadhi—Illumination (liberation) merging consciousness with God
Stage-7: Dhyana (Meditation)—Intense contemplation (a calm observance)
Stage-6: Dhaarana (Concentration)—fixing attention on single object
Stage-5: Pratyahar—Sense of withdrawal from external world and to go inward
Stage-4: Pranayama—Conscious-controlled, restrained yogic breathing (it will remove impure gas and extracts more oxygen in lungs)
Stage-3: Asana (Yogic posture)—Foundation of movement (It takes joints to full range, stretches soft tissues to its full length)
Stage-2: Niyam—Individual discipline (purity, contentment, austerity, study of God and soul, surrender to God)
Stage-1: Yama—Social discipline (nonviolence, nonlying (truth) non-stealing, sexual abstention/adultery, nonpossessiveness)

SEVEN CHAKRAS OF THE SUBTLE BODY

- Sahasrara: 1000 multicolored petals lotus situated at the top of skull. A state of pure consciousness—pituitary gland controls all endocrine glands functioning
- Ajna: Two violet colored petals located in the middle of forehead. Ida and Pingala Nadis merge with Shushumna with OM as syllable. It deals with consciousness and institution. Corresponding Pineal (light sensitive) gland produces melatonin which control sleep and awareness
- Vishuddhi: 16 pale blue petals located at throat near thyroid gland. The thyroxine hormone governs communication, and growth. Chakra controls independence
- Anahata: 12 green petals located near the heart and thymus gland. Gland governs immune system. Chakra controls circulation, unconditional love, passion, devotion

- Manipura: 10 yellow petals located near umbilicus, center of gravity. Adrenal glands govern digestion. Chakra controls personal power, expressiveness
- Swadhisthana: Six orange petals located in sacrum and correspond to testes and ovary which produces sex hormone for reproductive cycle. Chakra controls creativity
- Muladhar: Four red petals, located at the base of spine in the coccygeal region, relates to gonads and adrenal medulla. When survival is under threat it is for "fight or flight" response. Chakra governs stability, sexuality, sense of smell, security.

Dormant "Kundalini" rest at Muladhar chakra. Three nadis—Ida, Pingala, Shushumna, separate and make upward movement from here.

Yoga has many benefits which are scientifically explained. Muladhar is at the base of all chakras whereas anatomically, anal sphincter near muladhar chakra is a significant organ for determining the complete/incomplete spinal cord lesion.

Asana in yoga is similar to postures in physiotherapy as a foundation for motion. Also asana provide stretching of soft tissues and full range of motion to joints (generally in day to day activities we do not use joints to its full range). Similar exercises are done in physiotherapy.

Pranayama (with consciousness) are similar to breathing exercises. Meditation of mind eliminates worrying and conflicting thoughts takes brain to the "Alpha state": Brain becomes pure and pious and is well focused for assertive and affirmative thoughts for actions.

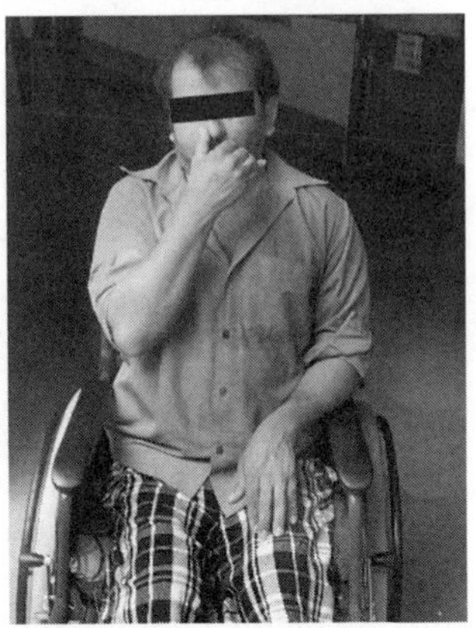

Fig. 1: A spinal cord injury patient doing ANULOM-VILOM pranayama

Some examples of the asanas which provide therapeutic effects

Paschimotasan—Patient is in long sitting and holding toes with fingers, where the spine and hips are in flexion and knees are in extension. The smoothly maintained, sustained posture breaks the extension spasticity-synergy and stretches hamstrings tightness in upper motor lesions.

Naukasan—Patient is in prone position, flexes both knees and holds toes with fingers, where the hips are in extension and knees are in flexion. Smooth-sustained posture provides, hip flexors stretching and breaking the spasticity-synergy.

Physiotherapist must take scientific measures before applying yoga practices to the patients.

KUNDALINI AWAKENING

"Kundalini Yoga consists of active and passive asana-based kriyyas, pranayama, and meditations which target the whole body system (nervous system, glands, and mental faculties, chakras) to develop awareness, consciousness and spiritual strength." -Yogi bhajan-Healthy, Happy, Holy Organization (3 HO).

Kundalini, a coiled up serpent like dormant spiritual energy or life force is located at the base of the spine near muladhar chakra (anal sphincter). During yogic breathing when Prana and Apana blend at the 3rd Manipur chakra, at naval, it initially drops down to the 1st and 2nd chakras before traveling up to the spine. The sleeping energy is awakened to travel along the Ida (left), Pingala (right) and Shushumna (center) Nadis and with organic energy it passes through 6 chakras and penetrate the 7th chakra or crown. It activates the Golden cord—the connection between the pitutary and pineal glands.

The majority of the physical postures focus on naval activity, activity of spine, and selective pressurization of the body points and meridians. Three bandhas—Mul bandh (closure of anal sphincter), Jalandhar bandh (tightening of lower abdominals) and Udian bandh (pressing chin to chest) three yogic locks and breathing in right and left alternate nostrils (Anulom-Vilom Pranayama). With Kapalbhati pranayam help to cleanse Nadis and pathways to help awaken Kundalini energy and travel from the muladhar chakra, going up towards shahasrara chakra.

KAPALBHATI PRANAYAMA

Kapal means forehead, *Bhati* means shining. This pranayama helps to get glow and luster on the face.

Sit in Padmasana or Sukhasana (crossed-leg sitting or available position). Placement of one hand on abdomen (Navel) helps to provide tactile cueing. Person will give emphasis on exhalation and the inhalation will be passive recoil (reverse of normal breathing where the exhalation is a passive recoil). Person exhales forcefully with a sudden and a sharp thrust with a simultaneous-strong lower abdominal contractions. Within a second this cycle should be completed and in a row initially 15–20 repetitions should be done and gradually it can be increased.

Benefits include—removal of residual air from lungs, clearing windpipe, lungs are strengthened, strengthening of lower abdominals, reduction in negative thoughts, reduction in blood pressure and blood sugar, removal of debris from mind (negative/conflicting thoughts), increasing the blood circulation, awakening of Kundalini with purity of mind, peace and pleasure.

It should be done with an empty stomach and person with hypertension should do it with lesser force and for less time. If person feels dizziness, discontinue it.

ANULOM-VILOM PRANAYAMA

Alternate nostril breathing: in crossed leg sitting (or any position) close left nostril with right ring and middle finger, slowly-smoothly-deeply breathe in through right nostril, hold breath for 5 seconds. Open left nostril and close right nostril with right thumb and slowly smoothly breathe out from left nostril, expiration is longer. Now reverse and repeat for 5 times. This improves gaseous exchange removing carbon dioxide and more oxygen to brain and body. It reduces respiratory and heart rates (Patient may practice any other pranayama). It is called Nadi Sodhan Pranayama in which all Nadis (tracts) are cleansed and cleared.

Scientifically—Pranayama is a conscious and controlled breathing (Restricting and Restraining) for a better gaseous waste removal and more extractions of oxygen for brain and body.

MEDITATION

For meditation, we have to use any one sensory organ and focus brain on one thing only for example, Looking constantly at a light (visual), Listening to the tic-tic-tic of wall clock (auditory), Chanting Lords name with "Rosary beads" (touch) (e.g. Swaminarayan), similarly slow down breathe and brain thoughts and consciously taste the food and smell the perfume.

"Vipasyana"—Nostril consciousness meditation technique. Sit in a crossed leg sitting position (or any position), close eyes, attention on nostrils. (Initially to develop habit, constantly see nostrils in the mirror). Repeatedly bring your attention on nostrils as brain will go away from nostril attention. Murmur in mind "nostrils-nostrils", slow down breath so as the coming out air get dispersed near nostrils. This will reduce the brain thoughts. Worrying and conflicting thoughts are eliminated and affirmative—assertive thoughts dominates. The brain will be cool and calm in an "Alpha state" with peace and pleasure for a purpose in life.

Lord Krishna suggested Arjuna in "Bhagvat Gita" to focus on nostrils for removing the depression due to grief of fighting with near and dear ones and to get focused for fighting. SCI patients need to be focused to fight for freedom.

"Savasana" (Sabasana) meaning making body like a "sab" (dead body). It is a "conscious" relaxation of the body. One has to relax body "consciously" and letting go the body organs starting from toes and going up to neck. Please remember that sleeping is not a Savasana. Consciousness is important.

SUN SALUTATION (SURYA NAMASKAR)

Useful for patient's partner and caregiver. It is a combination of "Posture and Motion" also worshipping Lord Sun, hence it integrates body-mind-soul with Divine. It stretches, strengthens joints and tissues. It provides physical strength, stamina and emotional equilibrium. There are 12 stages. It can be done anywhere but if done facing the Sun is better.

AYURVEDA

(Sanskrit language word—*Ayu* means Life, *Veda* means knowledge)

It is a Hindu traditional system of medicine with the "Shushruta and Charak Sanhita" as the text. The diagnosis is made by

- Akruti—appearance
- Nadi—pulse
- Sparsha—touch
- Jihva—tongue
- Druk—vision
- Shabda—speech
- Mutra—urine
- Mala—stool.

This system emphasize on good metabolism, good digestion, proper excretion. It focuses on yoga, meditation, exercises and sattvik (natural) diet. It believes in hygienic living with bath, clean teeth, skin care, eye washing.

Before starting with Ayurvedic medicines, the body is cleansed to remove toxins.

Purva karma—Prepurification before the "Panchkarma". Snehana is the whole body oil massage which will move the toxins to gastrointestinal tract. The soft tissue will become smooth and supple. It removes spasm and stress.

Swedan is the sweating of body by help of steam which removes toxins.

Panchkarma—Main five purification measures.

1. Vaman (Emesis therapy): Vomiting is carried out to remove mucus (Kapha) from the lungs
2. Virechana (Purgation therapy): A therapeutic laxative is done to remove excess bile (Pitta) from the gallbladder, liver and small intestine
3. Basti (Enema therapy): Introduction of herbal concoctions of sesame oil into the rectum to remove (Vata). It relieves constipation, distention, heart pain, chronic fever
4. Nasya (Herbal inhalation therapy): Inhalation of vapor of medicated herbs. It eliminates Kapha-oriented problems of ears, nose, throat, migraine, sinusitis, cataract, bronchitis
5. Rakta moksha: Bloodletting or small amount of blood extraction from vein. The disintegration of red blood cells in the liver leads to the formation of Pitta. If small amount of blood is extracted, a lot of tension is relieved that was created by Pitta. It also stimulates the spleen in order to produce antitoxin substances that can help to stimulate the immune system.

This system uses natural medical substances—cardamom, cinnamon, clove, etc. It is based on herbs, plants, flowers, fruits, vegetables. Herbal medicines are prepared for the treatment.

NATUROPATHY

(Naturo means nature, Pathy means disease)

It is based on the belief in "Vitalism", a special vital energy, Vital force which guides and regulates the life processes of metabolism, growth, adaptations, reproduction. It avoids the use of drugs or surgery. The treatment emphasizes on improving the life vitality by lifestyle modification with a natural life with house setup, cotton cloth; use of natural food, fruit, milk and curd; Flower essence; counseling for positivity and herbal medicines.

HOMEOPATHY

(Homeo means Like, Pathy means suffering)

Large doses of substances which cause symptoms can be used to treat those symptoms. German doctor Samuel Hahnemann in 1796 discovered this system of treatment. Along with him some volunteers did experiments on themselves and found that lower and smaller doses helped to reduce toxicity. The underlying causes of disease "Miasms" can be treated with Homeopathic medicines called "Remedies" are prepared with dilution in alcohol or distilled water and succession (vigorous shaking or striking on an elastic body). Homeopathy uses animal, plant, mineral and synthetic substances in its remedies, e.g. Arsenic oxide, Sodium chloride, Venom of the bushmaster snake, opium, Thyroid hormone. When prescribing medicines they use—Materia Medica—collections of "drug pictures" organized alphabetically by "remedy", Repertory—an index of disease symptoms.

ACUPRESSURE/REFLEXOLOGY

(Acu means needle, Pressure means to press)

It is similar to acupuncture principles. Acupressure uses pressure on specific pressure points with thumb or other body parts or blunt but pin-pointed objects.

The acupoints are located mainly in the palms and soles which are linked to all the body organs by Meridians lines. The first acupoint pressure creates a link with one collateral meridians and the respective body organ. The additional acupoint is pressed to reduce the blockage of flow of energy and stimulates organ.

It claims to be effective in nausea, vomiting, back pain, tension, headaches, and stomach pain and also to improve overall health with happiness.

Footwear, seat cushions are available to provide constant pressure.

ACUPUNCTURE

(Acu means needle, Puncture means to pierce in body with needle)

It is a Chinese system of treatment. The needles are made up of thin stainless steel which are flexible and are rustproof. They are disposable needles or if reused, they need to be sterilized to prevent contamination. The length varies from 13–130 mm. The longer are used for fleshy area and shorter for skinny area like face, ear.

The area is sterilized with alcohol then skillfully, the needle is inserted in a specific acupuncture point which correlates with qi meridians. Sometime needles are connected with a stimulator with a low voltage current which is passed for 10–60 minutes. Like acupressure, it will correct the blockage from the meridians and will connect the respective body organ for stimulation for better functioning.

MAGNETOTHERAPY

(Magneto means use of magnets, Therapy means treatment)

The earth is a big magnet with North and South poles. All body cells have magnetic fields. Practitioners believe that by applying the electrically charged permanent magnets on affected body parts, for 30–60 minutes, the magnets will restore the disturbed magnetic fields of the diseased cells.

Magnetic bracelets, magnetic jewelry, magnetic straps, magnetic cervical or lumbar belts, magnetic blankets, magnetic water is used to reduce the problem.

ASTROLOGY-HOROSCOPE-ZODIAC SIGNS-TAROT/ PSYCHIC-READING

These practitioners believe that it is a "Science of Stars". It is easy-to-learn it but takes long time to master it. All humans are curious to know about their course of life in future and the patients and their relatives seek services from astrology to get relief from the ailment.

Astronomy is the study of Sun, Stars, Moon, Planets and Galaxies in the space.

Astrology is the study of Sun, Moon and other Planets at the time of birth (not gestation) and their influence on person's personality, the future course of events including social, economical, medical, etc. These practitioners claim to get relief from problems with some rituals.

28

Speech Pathology and Audiology Services

Speech pathology: Patient's speech problems are evaluated and necessary speech therapy is provided to improve the speech and language.

Audiology: Hearing capacity of the patient is measured with an audiogram.

High cervical spinal cord injury patients, many a times have (TBI) traumatic brain injury and also due to spinal cord surgery, patients have speech problems of perception, prosodic, phonation and articulation.

DYSPHASIA (APHASIA)

A language disorder with problems of comprehension, production of speech and inability to read and write.

Global aphasia (both Sensory and Motor): Patient can speak and understand very little and can't read or write. Most severe aphasia.

Broca's aphasia (Motor): Patient can understand speech and the written words but speaking and writing is difficult. As patient understands but can not express, it is very frustrating for patient.

Wernicke's aphasia (Sensory): Patient speaks in gibberish (irrelevant speaking) but is not aware of it. Patient may have trouble in reading and writing.

Anomic aphasia: Patient understands speech and can read, but has difficulty finding words in speech and writing.

DYSPHAGIA

Dysphagia refers to disturbed deglutition (swallowing).

In spinal cord injury (SCI), patient may have traumatic brain injury (TBI), oral intubation, tracheostomy, spinal surgery, may have problems of swallowing. These patients are taught and trained how to do swallowing. In the beginning, liquid to semisolid to solid food for swallowing is given.

Vegetative functions training: ST and OT both work on this.

- Seeping fluid with lips
- Sucking the fluid with a straw
- Chewing food between teeth
- Swallowing.

Above functions are used for the eating and drinking. The same musculature is used for the production of voice and the speech.

Speech therapy

- Perceptions: Sensory inputs
  - Sight: Showing the actual people-places or people-places in the picture
  - Smell: Different odors and fragrance is given for smelling
  - Sound: Listening different sounds-high and low pitch
  - Touch: Informations of different objects with shape/size/texture/temperature
  - Taste: Taste training for sweet, sour, salty, bitter, umami
- Breathing to increase vital capacity and to improve control over breathing out
- Articulation: Vegetative function exercise.
  - Mouth exercises (Use mirror as feedback for all exercises)
    - Open mouth widely and close tightly
    - Jaw-side to side movement
  - Tongue exercises
    - Protrude tongue between lips
    - Sticking out tongue as far as you can
    - Tongue retraction and touching the roof of mouth—Place tongue behind your top teeth
    - Tip of the tongue to move on lip surface
  - Lip exercises
    - Lip protrusion and retraction
    - Lip press: Press lips tightly, hold for 5–10 seconds
  - Cheeks exercises
    - Fill cheeks with air, move air from one cheek to another
    - Fill cheeks with water and move water in the mouth
- Phonation: Repeatedly to practice to produce sounds
  - Vowels: a, e, i, o, u
  - Consonants: b, c, d, f, g, h.........z.
- Speech and language: To utter words, sentences with meaning

29

Occupational Therapy Service in the Ward and in the Department

Occupational therapist (OT) is a medical profession who plays an important role in the restoration, reshaping and rehabilitation of patients. Evaluation, intervention with outcome measures are their roles. With traditional and innovative activities, assistive devices, adaptation as tools, OT activates and assists in patient's activities to accomplish the aim. OT prepares patient for activities of daily living (ADL). Active participation in activities keeps the patient's mind engaged and patient is away from worries and depressive thoughts. OT have role to play in the settlement phase of Rehab—in the hospital setup and in the home setup.

OCCUPATIONAL THERAPY IN THE WARD

Patient is evaluated for the potential and problems and accordingly the OT program is planned.

- Upper limbs: Active movement and resisted work with a medicine ball
- Bed mobility: Active or assisted turning. When allowed sitting up, moving in the bed from one end to other
- Selfcare: Teaching and training them for brushing, bathing/sponging, dressing, shaving, grooming, feeding in lying or sitting position, assisted, if needed
- Transfers: From bed to wheelchair and from wheelchair to toilet and back. Transfer wooden boards are used, if needed (Fig. 1).

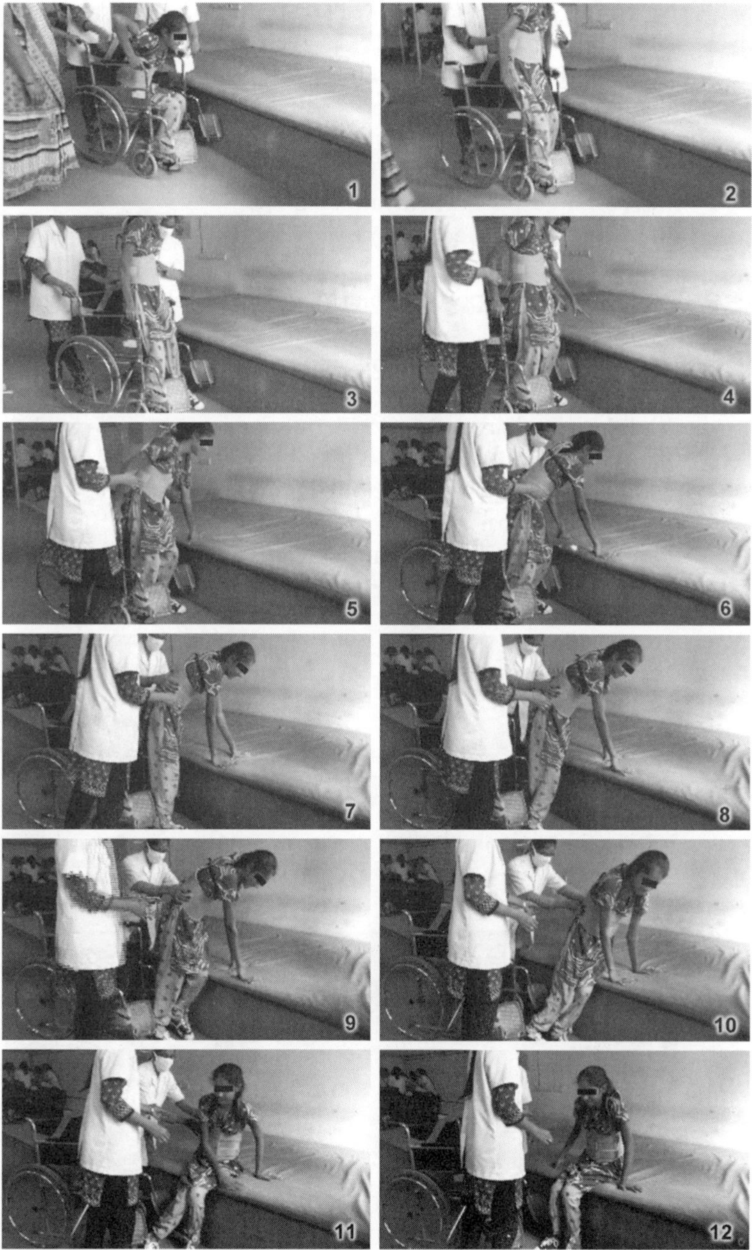

Fig. 1: A paraplegic patient transferring from wheelchair to high mat with minimal assistance

OCCUPATIONAL THERAPY IN THE DEPARTMENT

- Tilt table mobilization from 50° to 90°, with an increase of 5 degrees/day. During this, patients will do throwing and catching a ball activity
- Patients on wheel chair are gathered in the play area (Fig. 2)
  - Recreational sports are arranged daily
  - All patients are lined up in two rows facing each other and throw ball
  - Other individual sports are ball in the bucket, shot put, archery, Javelin throw
  - For pediatric patients, toy playing in the toy bank
  - Sanding—Vertical and horizontal sanding for upper limbs work
  - Traditional Indian-grain grinding stone moving for the working of upper limb work
  - Traditional Indian manual cloth thread making for the working of upper limb work
  - Standing in a frame and doing activities with upper limbs. Here lower limbs also works

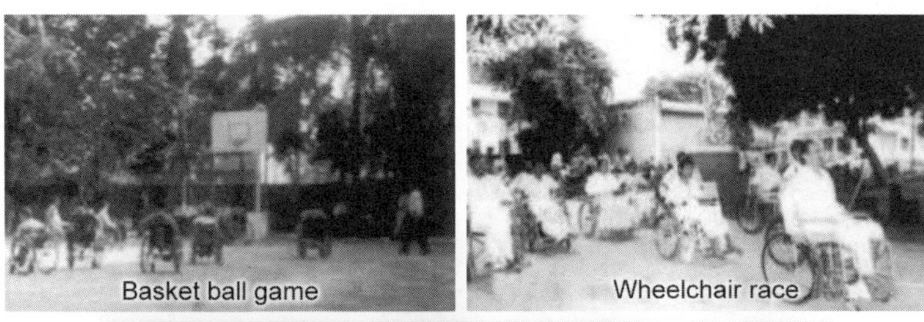

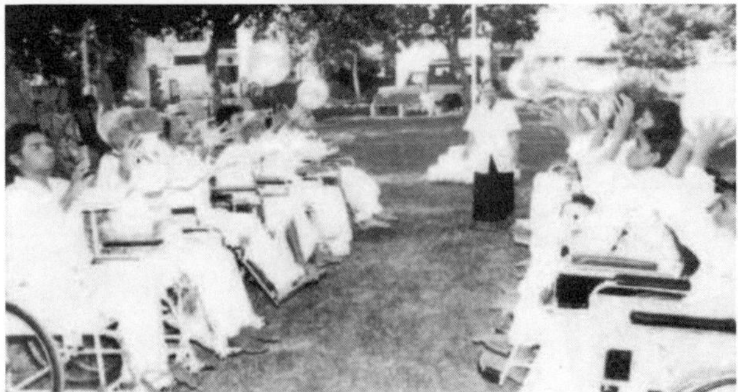

Fig. 2: Outdoor occupational therapy activities including sports

  - Creative activities like painting, knitting, tattoo making (Mehandi designs on hands/legs)
  - Fretsaw—Patient does craft work with hands, simultaneously moving lower limbs
  - Computer training for the educated patients.
- Adaptive devices are designed to facilitate the functions.
  - Spoon, brush, pen with a large ball type end of the handle, to improve grip
  - Tenodesis, long/short-opponens, knuckle bender splints to improve grip
  - Hand rails are fixed in toilet wall for an easy transfer to the toilet seats.
- Wheelchair management: Nearly 70% of SCI end up with a "Wheelchair life".
  - Patient is trained for a to and fro transfer, independent propulsion, turning, going up or down slopes and to go up or down on footpath/curb with "Wheelie" (learning to balance wheel chair on rear wheels with front wheels off the ground).
- Splinting: Simple splints are prepared for patient to reduce disability and to improve the activity.

30

Orthotic Services

Prosthesis replaces the lost body part, orthosis supports the weak part.

PROCEDURE

- Patient is evaluated with the muscle strength and other abilities, type of stump, etc.
- Rehabilitation team prescribes the necessary orthosis or prosthesis
- Orthosis-prosthesis is prepared in the workshop
- It is fitted and is checked by Ortho-Prostho bioengineers, orthopedics physiotherapists (PT) and occupational therapists (OT).
- Rigorous training is given in PT and OT department so as brain and body will accept it as body part, otherwise body will reject it and it will be useless.

Orthotic is a Greek word means to straighten or align is a specialty of medical engineering, concerned with the design, manufacture and applications of orthosis. It is used to:

- Control, guide, limit, immobilize joint or body segment
- Restrict movement in a given direction
- Assist movement
- Reduce weight-bearing forces
- Correct the shape and the functions.

Orthosis prescription is done by the group (Rehab round-OPD), prepared by the workshop, fitting checkup done by PT/OT/workshop, training is done in PT/OT dept.

- Rigid and Semirigid orthosis (Fig. 1)

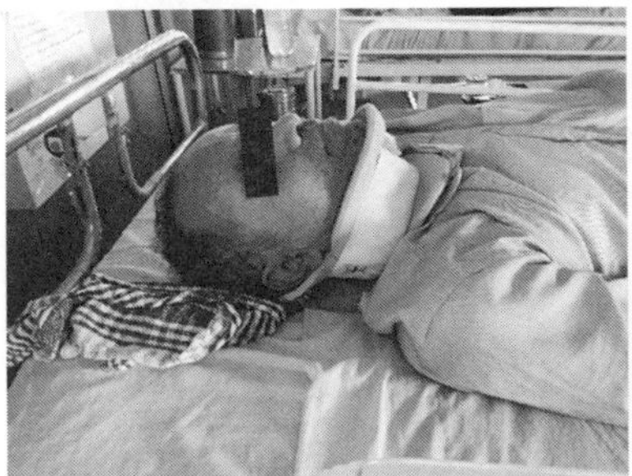
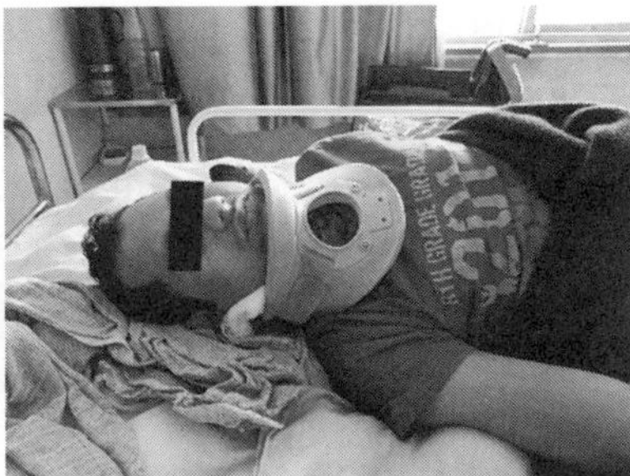

Fig. 1: Rigid and semirigid cervical orthosis

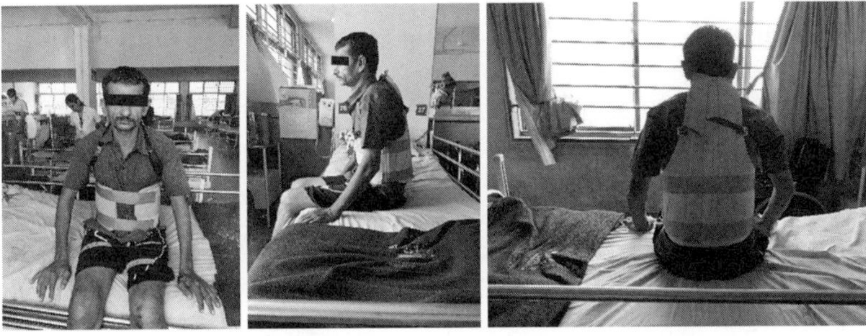

Fig. 2: Thoracolumbar spinal orthosis (Taylor's brace)

- SOMI—Sterno-occipital-mandibular immobilization that is what exactly it does for a rigid cervical immobilization. It is made up of aluminum and stainless steel
- Taylor's brace [Thoracolumbar Sacral Orthosis (TLSO)] is a light weight brace, covers dorsal, lumbar and sacral vertebrae; supports and immobilizes the spine in a neutral position, still permitting the required movement. Allows wearing and tightening of the brace by patient, no help from others (Fig. 2)
- LSO (Lumbosacral orthosis) holds the lumbar and sacral vertebrae in alignment
- Milwaukee orthosis is applied to correct the scoliosis of the spine
- HKAFO (Hip Knee Ankle Foot Orthosis) immobilizes hip, knee, ankle, foot hence the users adopts a "Swing to" or "Swing through" gait pattern with axillary crutches, which consumes lots of energy, can be used for indoor short distances (Fig. 3)

- KAFO (Scott and Craig Knee, Ankle, Foot orthosis) uses principle of Newton's third law of motion. The ankle is in slight dorsiflexion hence with "floor reaction force", patient keeps hip in hyperextension to maintain balance. The tautness of iliofemoral ligaments stabilizes the hips.

BENEFITS

- Easy to don (wear) and doff (remove)
- No hip joint or pelvic band
- Spreader bar controls the rotation and swing
- Laminated/Thermoplastic option
- Fast means of ambulations (4 and 2 point gait by hip hiking with the help of Quadratus Lumborum muscle) without undue energy expenditure.

AFO (Ankle-foot orthosis) Stabilizes ankle and foot, patient can walk with a stick. AFO with derotation bar applied during sleeping which also prevents leg rotation (Fig. 4).

TRS (Toe raising splint)—The spring/elastic between the calf and foot band, lifts the toes and foot to clear the ground when leg is flexed.

PKG (Posterior knee guard) is applied to prevent knee bending during walking.

Long-opponens splint: Hold the wrist in extension, thumb in opposition for grip.

Short-opponens splint: Thumb in opposition for grip.

Knuckle bender: In paralysis of lumbricals, splint bends MP joints and extends proximal IP joints, removes claw hand deformity for a good grip.

Tenodesis splint: Upon active wrist extension, with the help of the splint and the contracture of long flexors of fingers, patient can grip the object.

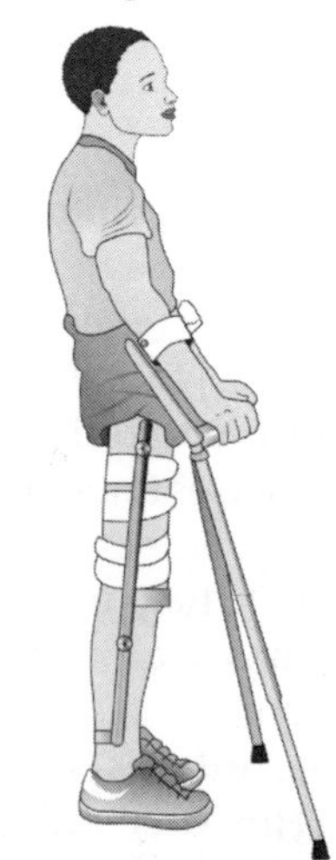

Fig. 3: A paraplegic patient standing with bilateral Hip Knee Ankle Foot Orthosis (HKAFO) and elbow crutches. (Note the hip and lumbar spine hyperextension attitude assumed by the patient)

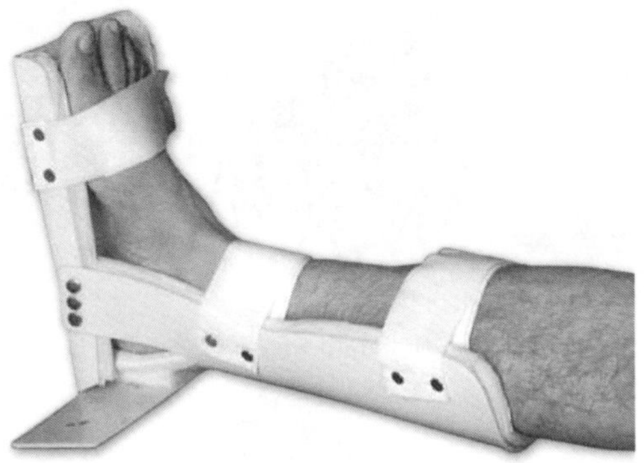

Fig. 4: Ankle-foot orthosis with derotation bar

FRO (Floor reaction orthosis): In polio patients with "0" muscle power in quadriceps, patient uses force from floor which is generated by the sole which is kept in 7°–8°of plantarflexion. The force will go up through the orthosis and will reach to the front of the knee and it will force the knee to go into the hyperextension to lock the knee (This is designed and developed by Dr Sethi, Orthopaedic surgeon of Jaipur, India).

The paraplegic AK Caliper is different from the traditional one in a way that there is no ischial seat weight bearing, as the paraplegics have sensory loss.

WHEELCHAIRS

Wheel chair (WC) of different designs and mechanism are available (Fig. 5)

- Manual self-propelled: They have large rear wheels with extruding hand rims so that the occupant can move and control the chair themselves. They have small front caster wheels for balance and wheels can rotate 360° for direction change. The chair has brakes, seat belts if needed, removable arm rests for an easy transfers-easy to access under the dining table, foot rest is swiveling. A cup holder is on one arm rest for placing the tea/ coffee/juice cup and a bag on other side to put needed materials, e.g. book (Fig. 6)
- Attendant propelled: They have handles on the back to push from behind

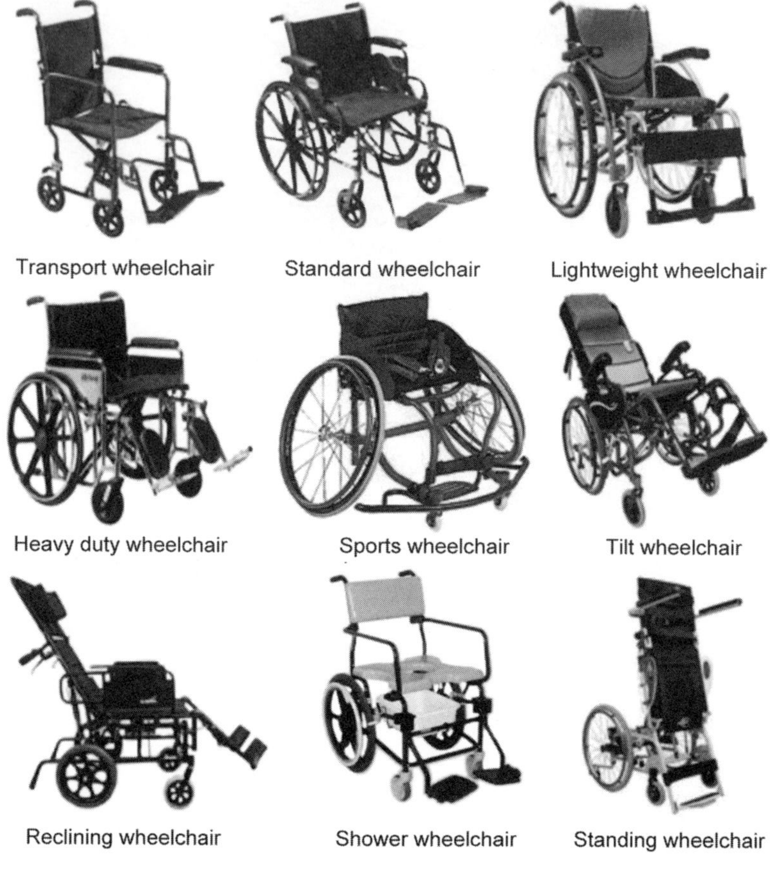

Fig. 5: Different kinds of wheelchairs

- Battery operated: The wheelchair is controlled with button. With more disability, Joy stick—a vertical handle that can move in two directions for control. Chin controlled—in C2–C3 lesion, the chair is controlled with chin movement. Pneumatic—Users use puff and sip air control for controlling the wheel chair
- Sports: Wheels are slanting inside at top, wide base, thin rim tyre.
- Reclining: The back rest can go back and down for comfort for heavy person, it distributes weight to prevent fall. Leg rests can also be lifted up resting with ease
- Pediatric: Smaller frames, narrowed seat, telescopic back handle to push or pull

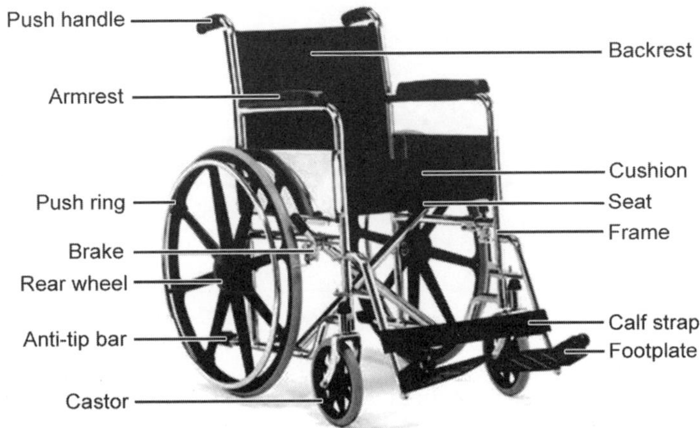

Fig 6: Components of standard wheelchair

- Heavy duty: Strong and sturdy for heavy person. Smaller rear wheels, not meant for self-propulsion. Reclined back rest to make sitting and transport easier
- Antibacterial: Treated with antibacterial technology on contact surfaces to prevent stain and odor causing bacteria. Upholstery is vinyl, not nylon
- MRI: Prepared from nonmagnetic material, e.g. PVC which prevent bacteria growth.

All wheelchairs can be folded, dismantled for an easy transportation in car.

CARE OF THE ORTHOTICS

- *Donning and doffing:* Wearing and removing training is given to the patient with minimum help from others. On first day, wear the orthosis for 1 hour. Remove and see the skin for red marks. If they do not fade away within 30 minutes, consult the Orthotist for realignment. Gradually increase the time and see the comfort
- *Cleaning and maintaining:* Apply spirit on metal to remove oil and dirt. Wipe with antibacterial towel. Do not clean it with water as this will harm the straps and metal fasteners. Keep orthosis away from heat, it will damage the plastic parts.

Similarly, prosthetic care is taken for durability and sustained satisfactory services.

31

Medical Social Worker's Services

Medical social worker is a medical professional. The professional has to undergo two years study program master in social work.

Medical social worker evaluates patient's medical, psychological, physical, social, economical problems and then moves to mobilize the resources, resolves issues, and finally brings resources (professional services and financial favors) to create an atmosphere near the patient to promote the rehab program.

- Coordinates all the resources as a liaison, for the welfare of the patient
- Counsels patient and caretakers about the problem, provide guidance as how to come out from it and boosts up the morale to cope up (Fig. 1)
- Educates patients and relatives about the body's functioning and about the spinal cord injury and how to prevent complications and promote progress in collaborations with Ortho, PT and OT
- Investigates issues which are hindering the rehab process
- Refers and assists patient, reaching to the needed resources

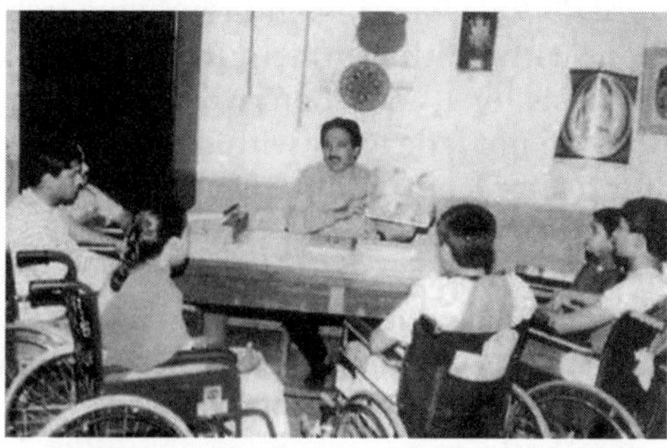

Fig. 1: Medical social worker counseling for social solutions

- Informs and assists patient about the benefits from government and other agencies
- Monitors, evaluates and records client's progress, according to the measurable goals described in the treatment plan
- Involves the non-government organization (NGO), according to the needs of a patient
- Visits patient's home with pysical therapy-occupational therapy (PT-OT) or gathers information about patient's house and home, prior to discharge and to do modification for removing the architectural barriers and to address the socio/economic issues
- Doorstep follow-up Safari program by Ortho, master of social work (MSW), PT, OT, P and O and nurse
- Disability screening medical camps, organized by Ortho, regional medical officers (RMO), MSW, PT, OT, P and O.

SOCIAL AND FAMILY PROBLEMS OF SCI

The SCI face many problems in the family and the society during and after the rehab process. The spouse thinking about the dark future is likely to leave patient and get divorced. Family and friends are eager and enthusiastic in the early phase of rehab but later on avoid assisting them, patients face mobility problems indoor and outdoor even if the architectural barriers are removed. Due to bladder-bowel problems and the incontinent accidents, they hesitate in taking part in the social events. People will not mix do them due to foul odor. If they are not earning, they will not get importance in the family in decision making and in day-to-day activities.

STEPS TOWARDS UNIVERSAL DESIGNS (FIGS 2 AND 3)

All the infrastructure facility be disabled friendly

- Houses with ramp, no thresholds between two rooms, Western toilets, railing in the toilets, bed and WC of same height, doors wide open for WC accessibility
- Roads must be smooth for WC/tricycle mobility (Fig. 2)
- Curb/footpaths with a slope at the end so as patients with WC or walking aids (e.g. crutches) can move up or down easily (simple solution with slanting slope)
- Public transportation—Bus with low floor for entry-exit
- Parking—Provision of a parking near the building entrance

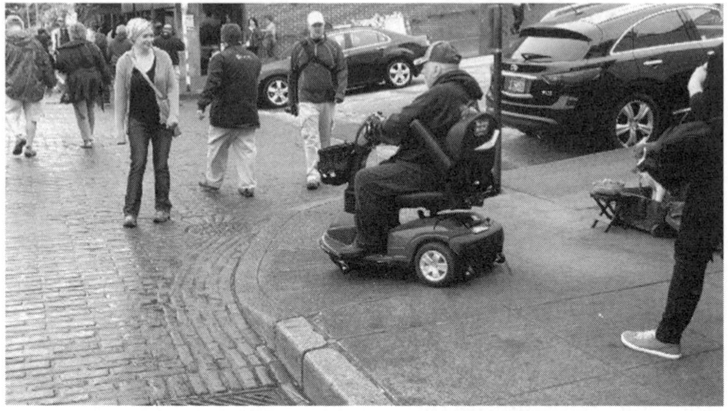

Fig. 2: Simple solution with slope

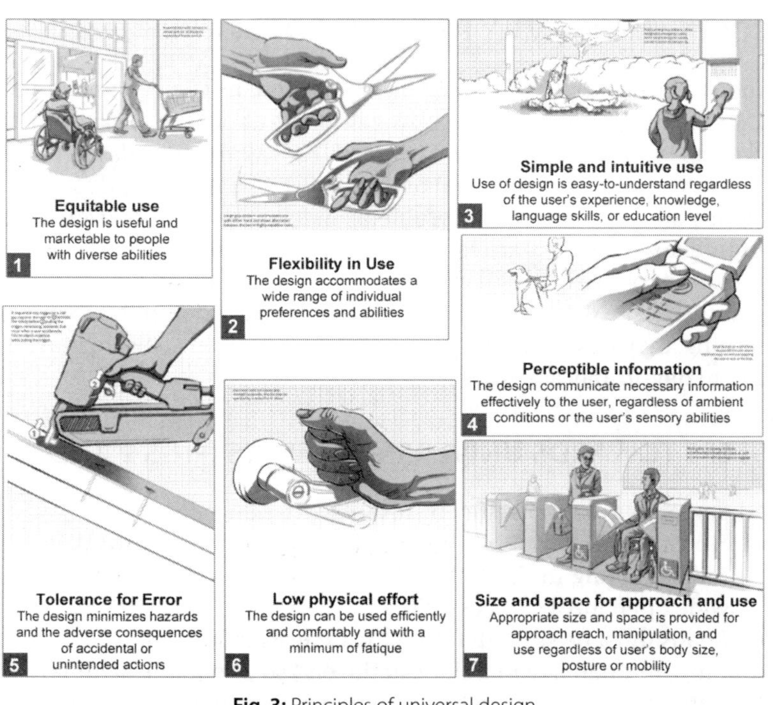

Fig. 3: Principles of universal design

- Public place—Facility of parking, ramp, wide doors, toilet accessibility.

ROLE OF NGO

Local and Global NGO

- Handicapped International (HI), UK based, Nobel Prize winner, works in over 60 countries
- A leg to stand on USA-based provide orthosis and prosthesis with Jaipur foot, Mahavir Viklang provide orthosis and prosthesis with Jaipur foot
- Red Cross
- Lions Club of Digvijaynagar—Asarwa, Satkarya Seva Samaj and other donors provide vocational aid to patients on discharge
- Kluge Children's Rehabilitation Center (KCRC), Kutchhi Rehabilitation Center
- Gujarat Sarvar Mandal help patients to get costly medicines free
- Jiv Daya trust of USA help patients in their rehab process.

Compared to Government, NGO have better local root level reality, small-simple network, quick decision making. When Government and NGO work together, better benefits reach to the patients. It was observed during earthquake of 2001 in Kutchh, India. The Government, efforts with local networking of the NGO gave excellent results. NGOs are helpful to support the patients and their relatives emotionally, socially and financially. They help to provide a home type atmosphere in the hospital. Involvement of NGO in the rehab process, encourage patients and enhance the program and they will be with them till they die.

CELEBRATION OF EVENTS

All human beings need enjoyment, appreciations and worth on earth with satisfaction and satiety in life which is also true for SCI. It is more important for patients who are struggling to survive had settled down. Such celebrations provide interaction with many people from different backgrounds of educations and earnings for caring and sharing with happy and harmonious moments. It takes

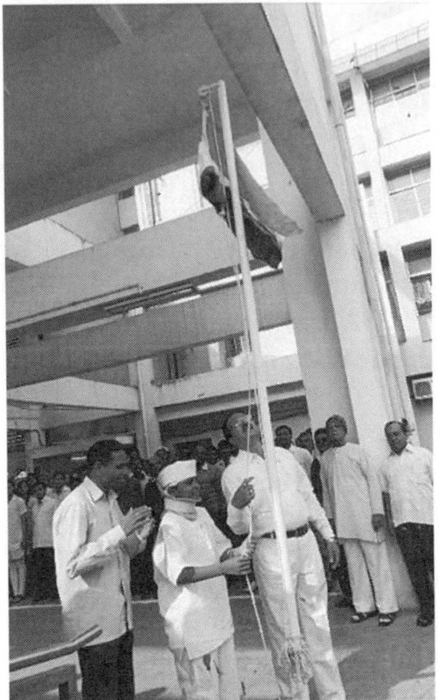

Fig. 4: A quadriplegic patient in flag hoisting program

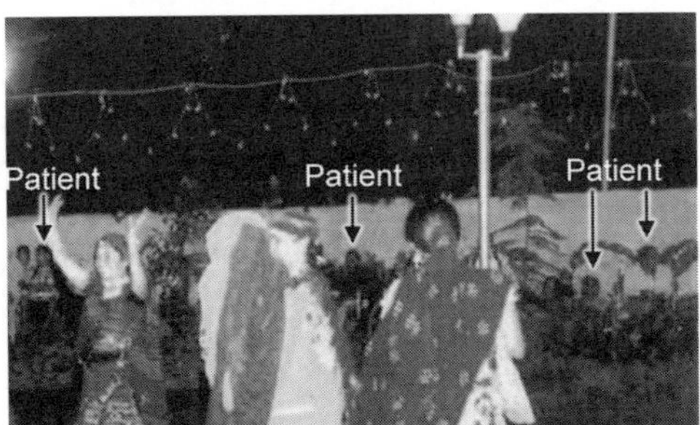

Fig. 5: Spinal cord injury patients attending a Navaratri celebration

patients away from the worries. Such variation in the day cycle remove monotony and boredom (Figs 4 and 5). Spinal cord injury patients should be encouraged to celebrate social and religious events like Rakshabandhan, Kite flying, "Gujarati Garba" dance during "Navaratri", Melodious musical concerts, magic show.

32

Sexual Alternatives for Patients and Partners

Spinal cord injury (SCI) patients are in general young adults. Sex is also their need and if not satisfied, can create mental problems which will hamper rehabilitation program. They are worried about it and face many problems for their sexual act. Patients need education and explanation about the sexual options. Psychologists, MSW, PT, OT arrange such lectures for them.

- Patient must realize that sex is possible with alternative methods
- Patient should start adjusting for sexual acts along with other Rehab programs
- Importance of personal hygiene and grooming for appealing appearance
- Communications and courtship with love making is needed for sexual act
- Some patients do not get orgasm but they do get sexual satisfaction
- Preparations before the act, they must clean the mouth and sexual organs. Use perfumes for a pleasant mood and deodorants to mask the foul odor
- Talking on sexual topics will bring patient and partner nearer with arousal
- Atmosphere—Dim light with erotic music can increase sexual fantasy.
- Foreplay—Kissing, hugging, patting, caressing genitals, gently biting each other and stimulation around rectal opening will help to achieve erection and sexual mood
- Vibrators are used, if patient lack hand dexterity
- Apply water soluble lubricant in vagina for an easy penetration of penis
- Orogenital stimulation—Patient may find more pleasure with this option, as the lips and tongue, which are not impaired by injury,

are more sensitive to touch and temperature than any other part of the body. In addition, the sensations received from the smell, taste and texture of partner's skin are powerful sex stimulants. Both are positioned (horizontal 69 position) in such a way that genitals are easily available to each other's mouth

- Oral therapy of Viagra approved by FDA (Foods and drugs administration-USA) in 1998, helps a SCI man to get greater rigidity and to sustain erection of penis for penetrations. It needs to be taken 60 minutes prior to the anticipated sexual act
- Intracavernosal injections of Papaverine help in satisfactory erection of penis for intercourse. With the training under the guidance of an urologist, male patient or partner can inject papaverine of their own
- Transurethral medication—A small pellet of Alprostadil is inserted transurethral under medical guidance, prior to the sexual act. It provides some rigidity but many men find burning sensation. It is not widely recommended
- Penile vacuum device—This device creates a vacuum around penis as a result blood is drawn in the corporal spaces. A band is placed at the base of the penis to maintain penile erection
- Penile implants—This usually is considered when other procedures have failed
  - Bendable implants are two plastic rods that are placed in the erection chambers of the space where blood gets accumulated during erection. It is less popular as the penis remains in permanent erection position
  - Inflatable implants consist of two cylinders that are surgically implanted into the penis. The pump is inserted into the scrotum. Upon squeezing the pump, the fluid (saline) will move to the cylinders and it makes the cylinders and the penis rigid. When deflated, the penis returns to a normal flaccid size (Hakim -2002)
- Male-female sexual toys for sexual gratifications
- Female SCI are given knowledge about child bearing and child birth
- Intercourse—Prolonged period of body adjustment is needed for sex act due to disability
  - Male patient, assumes lower position, the female partner is on top with her legs straddling on patient's body. This will have freedom of hip and pelvic movement

- Female patient, assumes lower position, the male partner plays dominant role for the rhythmic pelvic and hip movement
- Pelvis exercises will improve movements needed for sexual act
- Water bed—It serves double purposes. Firstly, it helps to prevent pressure sores, secondly, it helps in pelvic movements during coitus
- Problems and precautions—Bladder and bowel accidents are very common, hence cleaning towels and the air fresheners are to be kept handy.

• Sexual needs of "patient's partner". This is an important area which generally is not taken care of. Many partners are also adults; they are deprived of sexual act due to patient's disability and desires. It may take them to sexual adultery. Extramarital sex may strain marriage relationship and may hamper the rehab process and the quality of life. Partners are explained the dangers of sexual adultery and to avoid the sexual adultery they are taught alternative acts, e.g. erotic reading, erotic photo or video viewing and self help masturbation for the sexual gratification.

33

Vocational Counseling and Vocational Resettlement Services

VOCATIONAL TESTING AND VOCATIONAL TRAINING

Vocation/Occupation occupies a person for expressions, earning, enjoyment.

If a person is not working it creates problems. "An idle mind becomes devil's workshop." Spinal cord injury (SCI) in general are young adults, they have lots of energy, enthusiasm and dreams to do something and everything. After the survival stage and at the end of the settlement stage, once the patient has restored the physical potential, emotional equilibrium and independence in ADL, last stage of rehab is to train and to give a tool to the patient to earn the livelihood. Earnings give identity-image and independence, economic enhancement, social status, activity to remain active.

If vocationally patient is not settled, all our attainments will gradually go away and patient's activities will diminish, decay and complications will occur, giving morbidity, leading to mortality.

VOCATIONAL PROBLEMS OF SPINAL CORD INJURY

Vocation is an important aspect of a person, especially in their youth. Many SCI patients are young adults and the main bread earner of the family. Many are with less education doing physical work and not doing the office work. Majority of the patients can not return to their previous job and they need alternative arrangement.

- Vocational evaluation is done for physical potentials with disabling disability, education, aptitude, interest, special skills for earning (painting, knitting, craft, etc.)

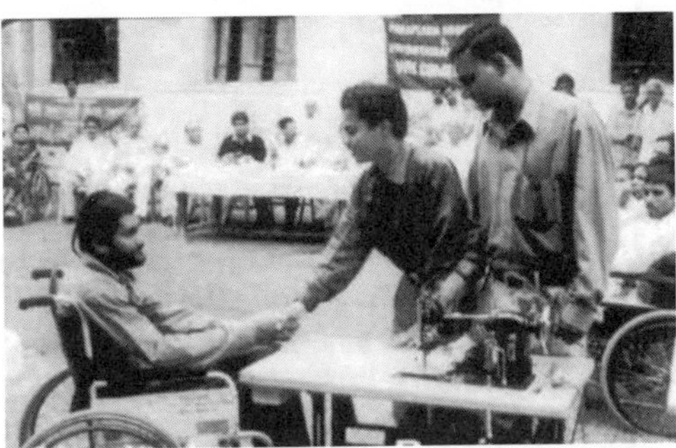

Fig. 1: A spinal cord injury patient receiving sewing machine from NGO

- Prevocational training—As per the patient's vocational potentials, social and surrounding situations, they are given training for the new vocation
- Vocational assistance—Benefits from Government/NGO including (e.g. 3% reservations in jobs) legal rights, initial material and money to start a self-employment business, e.g. sewing machine, readymade garments, cutlery items are given (Fig. 1).

Once they are ready for earning, necessary modifications are done to remove the architectural barriers at workplace to provide accessibility.

34

Discharge Plan

Before discharging the patient, it is essential to gather information about the infrastructure facility of the house and the surroundings for the accessibility. Needful modification should be done to remove architectural barriers. Arrangements for family integration, social support, and financial favors are also taken care of.

Independence in day-to-day activities is measured before discharge.

BARTHEL INDEX

It is the most simple scale and most suitable for spinal cord injury (SCI). In 1965, the scale was introduced and it has been modified twice. It uses 10 variables, describing activities of daily living (ADL) and mobility, it has 0–20 score and higher score indicates greater independence. The amount of physical assistance and time needed to perform the task is considered. Information can be gathered from patient's self-report, from a person familiar with patient or by observations.

- Bowels:
  - 0-Incontinent
  - 1-Occasional accident (1/week)
  - 2-Continent
- Bladder:
  - 0-Incontinent or catheterized
  - 1-Occasional accident (1/24 hours)
  - 2-Continent for over 7 days
- Toilet use:
  - 0-Dependent
  - 1-Needs some help

    - 2-Independent wiping, dressing
- Bathing:
    - 0-Dependent
    - 1-Independent in shower
- Grooming:
    - 0-Needs help
    - 1-Independent face/hair/teeth/shaving
- Dressing:
    - 0-Dependent
    - 1-Half unaided
    - 2-Independent buttons, zips
- Feeding:
    - 0-Unable
    - 1-Needs help cutting, etc.
    - 2-Independent (food within reach)
- Transfers:
    - 0-Unable, no sitting balance
    - 1-(1–2 person help)
    - 2-Minor help—3-Independent
- Mobility:
    - 0-Immobile
    - 1-WC independent
    - 2-Walks with help of 1 person
    - 3-Independent but may use a stick
- Stairs:
    - 0-Unable
    - 1-Needs help for aid
    - 2-Independent up and down.

FUNCTIONAL INDEPENDENCE MEASURE

Functional independence measure (FIM) assesses physical and cognitive disability. It consists of two subscales—motor and socio-cognitive. FIM is not SCI specific. It has limitations and ceiling effect with the socio-cognitive subscale for individuals with SCI and it does not measure the social, psychological or vocational impact of disability experienced by SCI.

FIM is completed by observations of performance. The motor subscales includes 13 items:

1. Eating

2. Grooming
3. Bathing
4. Dressing-upper
5. Dressing-lower
6. Toileting
7. Bladder management
8. Bowel management
9. Bed to chair transfer
10. Toilet transfer
11. Shower transfer
12. Locomotion—ambulations or wheelchair
13. Stairs.

Socio-cognitive subscale includes 5 items

Comprehension, expression, social interaction, problem solving, memory

The scoring is as follows:

- No helper required:
  - 7—complete independence, 6—Modified independence—Use of device but no physical assistance
- Helper modified dependence
  - 5—Supervision or setup, 4—Patient performs 75% and minimum contact assistance, 3—Patient performs 50-74% and moderate assistance
- Helper with complete dependence
  - 2—Patient performs 25-49% and maximal assistance, 1—Patient performs less than 25% and total assistance, 0—Activity does not occur.

SPINAL CORD INDEPENDENCE MEASURE (SCIM)

SCIM III was developed in 2002 as a modification of the two previous one. The SCIM I and II were found to be valid and reliable but did not take into account of intercultural differences. SCIM III has been developed, validated and found to be highly reproducible for SCI.

SCIM has three specific areas:

1. Self-care including bathing, dressing, grooming, feeding (score 0-0)
2. Respiration, bladder, bowel management and use of toilet (score 0-40)

3. Mobility ability—bed mobility, transfers, indoor-outdoor mobility (score 0–40).

WALKING INDEX FOR SPINAL CORD INJURY

Walking index for spinal cord injury (WISCI) is a measure of ambulations (10 meters) designed specifically for SCI. The score is from 0 to 20. Level 0, patient is unable to stand and/or participate in walking. Level 20, patient ambulates with no devices, may be with brace and no assistance.

On discharge

- Patient and relatives are given necessary information and instructions.
  - Precautions to prevent problems, e.g. pressure sores, contractures, respiratory dysfunction, urinary tract infection (UTI), to protect anesthetic limbs from hot and sharp objects
  - They are taught some simple exercises.
- Patients are encouraged to come for follow-up in the rehab OPD
- SCI safari is arranged for doorstep follow-up at their home.

35

Follow-up Care—A Lifelong Care

Spinal cord injury (SCI) is a lifelong problem and the patients die due to the complications. For better quality of life they need a regular check up by the rehab team.

It is observed that the patient after discharge were finding it difficult to come for a follow-up in the rehab OPD of the Institute due to the problems of finances, social, transportation, 2–3 persons as escorts as well as extreme handicap. Due to this, there were a large number of patients who were coming for readmission with preventable causes, if they had come for follow-up.

SCI SAFARI PROGRAM

"Dennis Burkitt's Tumor Safari concept"—a Safari project is started since 1984 for doorstep follow-up. A team of Ortho, PT, OT, P and O, MSW and a nurse visit rehabilitated discharged patients at the doorstep in their own living place in a Safari van (Fig. 1).

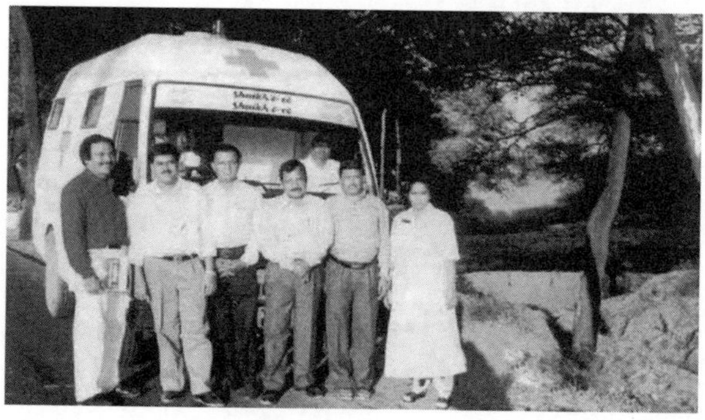

Fig. 1: Safari team

The patients are helped on the spot in the form of evaluation of the status of patient by each professional, after then necessary measures are taken. Necessary medications are given, dressing is done if there is a pressure sore and dressing material is also given. PT/OT teach stretching, strengthening and ADL exercises. P and O will do repair or replacement for the orthosis and mobility aid. Vocational counselor will give guidance and help for the vocational issues. MSW gives information of the nearby medical and rehab services.

36

Rehabilitation: Resources and Rhythm for Spinal Cord Injury in USA

TRANSPORTATION OF PATIENTS WITH SPINAL CORD INJURY

The patient with an acute SCI are expeditiously and carefully transported from the site of injury to the nearest capable definitive care medical facility. The modes of transportation chosen are based on the patient's clinical circumstances, distance from target facility, and geography to be traveled and should be the most rapid means available (Ambulance, Helicopter Service, etc). Immobilization of patients with acute cervical spinal cord and/or spinal column injuries is recommended. Cervical SCIs have a high incidence of airway compromise and pulmonary dysfunction; therefore, respiratory support measures should be available during transport.

At the accident scene, emergency personnel will immobilize the head and neck to prevent movement, put a rigid collar around the neck, and carefully place the person on a rigid backboard to prevent further damage to the spinal cord. Sedation may be given to relax the person and prevent movement. A breathing tube may be inserted if the injury is to the high cervical cord and the individual is at risk of respiratory arrest.

EMERGENCY ROOM MANAGEMENT OF SPINAL CORD INJURY

At the hospital or trauma center, realigning the spine using a rigid brace or axial traction (using a mechanical force to stretch the spine and relieve pressure on the spinal cord) is usually done as soon as possible to stabilize the spine and prevent additional damage.

Fractured vertebrae, bone fragments, herniated discs, or other objects compressing the spinal column may need to be surgically removed. Spinal decompression surgery to relieve pressure within the spinal column also may be necessary in the days after injury. Results of a neurosurgical study shows that, in some cases, earlier surgery is associated with better functional recovery.

Physicians determine the level and extent of the injury by using x-rays, MRIs, or CT scans. The patient will also undergo a thorough neurological examination. This measures sensation, muscle tone and reflexes of all limbs and the trunk. The results will be reflected in what is called an American Spinal Injury Association (ASIA) classification of spinal cord injury scale, a tool used to classify the spinal cord injury patient into various categories (ASIA A, B, C, D, or E; A is the most impaired, E the least). During an ASIA exam, the physician looks at the variety of determinants, such as muscle movement, range of motion, and notes whether or not the person can feel light touch or sharp and dull sensations.

HOW ARE SPINAL CORD INJURIES CLASSIFIED?

Once the swelling from within and around the spinal cord has eased a bit—usually within a week to 10 days—physicians will conduct a complete neurological exam to classify the injury as complete or incomplete. An incomplete injury means that the ability of the spinal cord to convey messages to or from the brain is not completely lost. People with incomplete injuries retain some sensory function and may have voluntary motor activity below the injury site. A complete injury prevents nerve communication from the brain and spinal cord to the parts of the body below the injury site. There is a total lack of sensory and motor function below the level of injury, even if the spinal cord was not completely severed. Studies have shown that people with incomplete injuries have a greater chance of recovering some function in the affected limbs than those with a complete injury.

CAUSES OF SCI IN US (TRAUMATIC CAUSES)

Incidence and Statistical Data

Vehicle crashes are the leading cause of injury, followed by falls, acts of violence (primarily gunshot wounds), and sports.

The National SCI database is a prospective longitudinal multicenter study that captures data from an estimated 13% of new SCI cases in the US from 28 federally funded SCI Model Systems since 1973.

Incidence

It is estimated that the annual incidence of SCI, not including those who die at the scene of the accident, is approximately 40 cases per million population in the US or approximately 12,500 new cases each year, given the current population size of 313 million people in the US.

Prevalence

The number of people in the US who are alive in 2014 who have SCI has been estimated to be approximately 2,76,000 persons, with a range from 2,40,000 to 3,37,000 persons. The average age at injury has increased from 29 years during 1970s to 42 years since 2010.

Gender and Race/Ethnicity

Approximately 79% of spinal cord injuries occur among males. Currently, about 24% of spinal cord injuries occur among blacks, which is higher than the proportion of blacks in the general population (12%).

Neurologic Level and Extent of Lesion

The most frequent neurologic category is incomplete tetraplegia followed by incomplete paraplegia, complete paraplegia, and complete tetraplegia. Less than 1% of persons experienced complete neurologic recovery by hospital discharge.

Marital Status

More than half of persons with SCI are single/never married when injured. The percentage of persons who are married slowly increases as the years postinjury increase, as does the divorce rate.

Education

Over half of persons with SCI are high school graduates at the time of injury. Level of education slowly increases over postinjury years.

Occupational Status

At one year after injury, 12% of persons with SCI are employed, and by 20 years postinjury, about one third are employed.

Hospital Stay Days

Length of stay days hospitalized in the acute care unit have declined from 24 days in the 1970s to 11 days since 2010. Substantial downward trends are also noted for days in the rehabilitation unit (from 98 to 36 days).

Rehospitalization

About 30% of persons with SCI experience one or more hospitalizations during a 12-month period. Among those rehospitalized, the length of hospital stay averages about 23 days. Diseases of the genitourinary system are the leading cause of rehospitalization, followed by disease of the skin. Respiratory, digestive, circulatory, and musculoskeletal diseases are also common causes.

Lifetime Costs

The average yearly health care and living expenses and the estimated lifetime costs that are directly attributable to SCI vary greatly according to severity of injury. These figures do not include any indirect costs, such as losses in wages, fringe benefits, and productivity which average $70,849 per year in November 2013—but vary substantially based on education, severity of injury, and preinjury employment history.

Life expectancy is the average remaining years of life for an individual. Life expectancies for persons with SCI are still significantly below life expectancies for those without SCI and have not improved since the 1980s.

Mortality rates are significantly higher during the first year after injury than during subsequent years, particularly for severely injured persons.

Cause of Death

Persons enrolled in the National SCI database since its inception in 1973 have now been followed for 40 years after injury. During that time, the causes of death that appear to have the greatest impact on reduced life expectancy for this population are pneumonia and septicemia. There has been no change in the mortality rate for septicemia in the past 40 years, and only slight improvement in mortality due to respiratory diseases.

This is a publication of the National Spinal Cord Injury Statistical Center, Birmingham, Alabama, (Grant Number H133A110002), and the Model Systems Knowledge Translation.

EMERGENCY MANAGEMENT

Today, improved emergency care for people with spinal cord injuries, antibiotics to treat infections, and aggressive rehabilitation can minimize damage to the nervous system and restore function to varying degrees. Advances in research are giving doctors and people living with SCI hope that spinal cord injuries will eventually be repairable. With new surgical techniques and developments in spinal nerve regeneration, cell replacement, neuroprotection, and neurorehabilitation, the future for spinal cord injury survivors looks brighter than ever.

STABILIZATION

Once a person is injured, the first priority is to stabilize the patient's breathing, blood pressure and spinal column (in most cases using a back board and a cervical neck collar). A patient with a suspected SCI will most likely be brought to or moved to the nearest Level 1 Trauma Center, which provides the highest level of surgical care to trauma patients, with a full range of specialists and equipment available 24 hours a day.

During the early days of hospitalization, a variety of medications may be used to control the extent of the damage to the spinal cord, alleviate pain, treat infections, and other issues related to the injury. Patients may be sedated and put into traction to prevent further damage. Some other types of traction techniques are metal bracing attached to weights or a body harness, a halo to prevent the head from moving, or a rigid neck collar.

NEUROPROTECTION

These therapies, also called neuroprotective therapies, aim to stop or reduce the immediate responses (such as swelling) to the injury that may further lead to spinal cord damage. Methylprednisolone is a steroid drug sometimes used in the first few hours after an injury; it is intended to reduce inflammation and improve recovery but there is no clear evidence to support this. Still, it is commonly used though it may not be appropriate in all cases.

Therapeutic hypothermia (spinal cord cooling) is a medical treatment that lowers the body temperature in order to protect the cells in the body from damage after a traumatic brain or spinal cord injury, stroke or cardiac event. Body temperature can be lowered by invasive methods, using catheters filled with saline to cool a patient's blood as it leaves the heart, thus lowering the temperature of the whole body. Noninvasive techniques use special blankets that have cold water running through them. These blankets may be combined with ice packs or cold fans in order to achieve more rapid temperature decline. The use of local therapeutic hypothermia at the time of surgery appears safe but no criteria for treatment guidelines have been established.

Surgical Interventions

Once a patient is medically stable, he or she will meet with a surgeon to make the decision on surgical interventions. Surgery is recommended for many reasons, such as removal of bone fragments, foreign objects, blood clots, herniated disks, fractured vertebrae, spinal tumors or anything that appears to be compressing the spine. Surgery to stabilize the spine helps prevent future pain or deformity.

Surgical Stabilization

Stabilization of the spinal cord is a common surgical intervention following a spinal cord injury. This procedure removes bone fragments and restores the alignment of the vertebrae, thus reducing compression on the spinal cord. Stabilization can occur within the first 72 hours or it may be delayed until after the body has been medically stabilized. There is no evidence to support an advantage for either early or delayed treatment.

Spinal Fusion

If the vertebrae in the spinal column appear unstable, the doctor may perform a spinal fusion. A spinal fusion may be done with metal plates, screws, wires and/or metal rods; sometimes small pieces of bone from other areas of the body (usually the hip or knee) or from a cadaver (bone bank) are used. Bone grafts help the patient's bones grow, thus serving to fuse the vertebrae. In cervical injuries, the stabilization can be done through the throat (anterior) or through the neck (posterior) or both. Thoracic and lumbar injuries are usually approached through the back.

RESPIRATORY

The lungs themselves are not usually affected by paralysis but the muscles of the chest, abdomen, and diaphragm may be. If complete paralysis occurs at level C3 or above, the phrenic nerve is no longer stimulated and the diaphragm will not function. Some individuals with lower level injuries may also need ventilator assistance for short periods of time before they can breathe on their own (called being weaned off the ventilator). Successful weaning from a ventilator is impacted by many factors: age, level of injury and time spent on the ventilator.

People injured at the mid-thoracic level or higher may have trouble taking deep breaths and exhaling forcefully. This can lead to lung congestion and respiratory infections. Ways of preventing respiratory complications include maintaining proper posture, coughing regularly (if necessary, with assistance), following a healthy diet, drinking plenty of fluids, eliminating smoking or being around smoke, exercising, and getting vaccinated for influenza and pneumonia.

STEM CELL TREATMENT FOR SPINAL CORD INJURY

Beike's stem cells have been used to treat patients diagnosed with spinal cord injury since 2005. The aim of the treatment is to regenerate the nerve cells that were damaged in patient's spinal cord after the original injury by using stem cell transplantation. To do so, stem cells are injected in great quantity through IVs and lumbar punctures in order to better target the damaged area.

Optionally and in addition to stem cell transplantation, a cutting edge epidural stimulation technology is provided that helps electrical signals to bypass the injury site, thus easing the communication between the brain and body parts below the injury.

Before considering stem cell therapy and epidural stimulation, the patient should have undergone any surgery recommended by local doctors, such as spine decompressive surgery.

REHABILITATION

How does rehabilitation help people recover from spinal cord injuries?

No two people will experience the same emotions after surviving a spinal cord injury, but almost everyone will feel frightened, anxious, or confused about what has happened. It is common for people to have very mixed feelings: relief that they are still alive, but disbelief at the nature of their disabilities.

Rehabilitation programs combine physical therapies with skill-building activities and counseling to provide social and emotional support. The education and active involvement of the newly injured person and his or her family and friends is crucial.

A rehabilitation team is usually led by a doctor specializing in physical medicine and rehabilitation (called a physiatrist), and often includes social workers, physical and occupational therapists, recreational therapists, rehabilitation nurses, rehabilitation psychologists, vocational counselors, nutritionists, a case worker, and other specialists.

In the initial phase of rehabilitation, therapists emphasize regaining communication skills and leg and arm strength. For some individuals, mobility will only be possible with the assistance of devices, such as a walker, leg braces, or a wheelchair. Communication skills, such as writing, typing, and using the telephone may also require adaptive devices for some people with tetraplegia.

Physical therapy includes exercise programs geared toward muscle strengthening. Occupational therapy helps redevelop fine motor skills, particularly those needed to perform activities of daily living, such as getting in and out of a bed, self-grooming, and eating. Bladder and bowel management programs teach basic toileting routines. People acquire coping strategies for recurring episodes of spasticity, autonomic dysreflexia, and neurogenic pain.

Vocational rehabilitation includes identifying the person's basic work skills and physical and cognitive capabilities to determine the likelihood for employment; identifying potential work places and any assistive equipment that will be needed; and arranging for a user-friendly workplace. If necessary, educational training is provided to develop skills for a new line of work that may be less dependent upon physical abilities and more dependent upon computer or communication skills. Individuals with disabilities that prevent them from returning to the workforce are encouraged to maintain productivity by participating in activities that provide a sense of satisfaction and self-esteem, such as educational classes, hobbies, memberships in special interest groups, and participation in family and community events.

Recreation therapy encourages people with SCI to participate in recreational sports or activities at their level of mobility, as well as achieve a more balanced and normal lifestyle that provides opportunities for socialization and self-expression.

Adaptive devices may also help people with spinal cord injury to regain independence and improve mobility and quality of life. Such devices may include a wheelchair, electronic stimulators, assisted gait training, neural prostheses, computer adaptations, and other computer-assisted technology.

Robotics and Spinal Cord Injury

Despite a lack of evidence for the use of UE robotics in the population with SCI, several studies have been completed on the use of robotics to elicit lower-extremity (LE) motor return in patients with incomplete SCI. These studies are based on the Central Pattern Generator Theory (Grillner, 1979, 1985; Pearson and Rossignol, 1991). According to the theory, repetitive movements can stimulate motor recovery even in the absence of complete central nervous system innervation. Central pattern generators consist of relatively small and autonomous neural networks that, when stimulated during specific repetitive movements, can produce rhythmic movement patterns, even in the absence of motor and sensory feedback from the arms or legs (Barrie`re, Leblond, Provencher, and Rossignol, 2008).

Implications for Occupational Therapy Practice

The results of this study have the following implications for occupational therapy practice:

- Upper-extremity robotics is a beneficial tool that can be used in combination with traditional occupational therapy for treating UE dysfunction in the SCI population

- Incorporating new technology in occupational therapy treatment is important to the evolution and progression of our field.

Environmental Control Units

Environmental control units (ECUs) are devices that have the potential to help persons with quadriplegia independently control electronic items at home, work, or school. ECUs can aid these persons in using the telephone, controlling the television, switching lights on and off, running appliances or computers, and managing the front door and house temperature. They also provide a sense of safety by enabling the person to summon help independently. Thus, ECUs provide a way for persons with severe disabilities to participate in life activities that would otherwise not be possible, giving them greater independence and enhanced quality of life (Garrison, 1982; Vanderheiden, 1982).

Environmental control units consist of a control interface or input device (e.g. keyboard, joystick, switch, voice activator) and a feedback display that reflects the action being controlled (Cook and Hussey, 1995). The control interface and user display are connected to a processor that produces the activity output. The four basic types of signal transmission are ultrasound, infrared light, radiofrequency waves, and house wiring (alternating current power line). The activity output provides independent control over the electrically powered devices.

WHAT RESEARCH IS BEING DONE?

Scientists continue to investigate new ways to better understand and treat spinal cord injuries.

Much of this research is supported by the National Institute of Neurological Disorders and Stroke (NINDS), a part of the National Institutes of Health (NIH). Other NIH components, as well as the Department of Veterans Affairs, other federal agencies, research institutions, and voluntary health organizations, also fund and conduct basic to clinical research related to improvement of function in paralyzed individuals.

Many hospitals have developed specialized centers for spinal cord injury care. Many of these bring together spinal cord injury researchers from a variety of disciplines for partnerships regarding basic and clinical research, clinical care, and knowledge translation.

Current research is focused on advancing our understanding of four key principles of spinal cord repair:

- Neuroprotection—protecting surviving nerve cells from further damage
- Regeneration—stimulating the regrowth of axons and targeting their connections appropriately
- Cell replacement—replacing damaged nerve or glial cells
- Retraining CNS circuits and plasticity to restore body functions.

Neuroprotection

Strategies involving neuroprotection are aimed at preventing cell death, limiting or reducing inflammation, and stopping over-excitability of certain cells and their functions. Investigators are looking at ways to reduce inflammation within or near the injured spinal cord, which can restrict blood flow, affect nerve signal transmission, and increase cell death.

One approach is using steroid drugs to reduce nerve cell damage and suppress activities of immune cells. One clinical trial identified slight improvement in motor function among some individuals who were given a steroid within 8 hours after injury. However, other trials showed the drug's modest benefit did not outweigh serious side effects. Steroid therapy has not been approved by the US Food and Drug Administration (FDA) for the treatment of acute spinal cord injury.

Antibiotics, which can cross the protective blood-brain barrier, have been shown to improve motor function, restoration, decrease lesion size, and reduce cell death in animal models of SCI.

The kidney hormone erythropoietin promotes the growth of new red blood cells and increases oxygen levels in the blood. Studies in animal models have shown that erythropoietin can reduce inflammation in the brain, improve blood flow to the brain, and reduce nerve cell death following brain injury. It also aids in the recovery of motor function. However, other trials in animal models show conflicting results regarding the drug's usefulness in preventing inflammation and cell death. Researchers continue to study the drug in preclinical models.

Therapeutic hypothermia (controlled lowering of the body's core temperature) can protect cells from damage following cardiac arrest, stroke, and traumatic brain injury. Therapeutic hypothermia has been shown to reduce the swelling and inflammation that presses on the spinal cord following injury in animal models and in small, limited human studies. It can also reduce damage to susceptible neurons following the primary injury, reduce damage to spinal cord microvasculature, and improve functional outcome. Researchers are studying the safety and effectiveness of different durations of hypothermia following spinal cord injury.

Researchers are trying to manipulate macrophages—a type of white blood cell that travels to the injury site during the inflammatory response—to promote nerve cell growth without causing further tissue damage. Following a spinal cord injury, macrophages at the site of injury begin to remove cellular debris and receive signals that help them promote the growth of axons. But, within a few days postinjury, the collection of macrophages increases inflammation, scarring, and toxicity, which can worsen the damage. Scientists hope to learn how to signal macrophages to continue their restorative function while turning off their damaging consequences.

The buildup of sodium and glutamate in cells following a spinal cord injury can lead to cell damage and impaired or blocked cell signaling. The drug riluzole, which slows the progression of the disease amyotrophic lateral sclerosis, has shown in animal models to improve motor function and reduce cell death loss caused by decreased blood flow following spinal cord injury. The experimental drug HP 184 blocks the entry of sodium into cells (which can impair nerve function) and may enhance cell signaling in surviving axons that have had their protective myelin cover either destroyed or damaged following spinal cord injury. Other scientists are examining drugs that target glutamate, whose release is greatly increased following a spinal injury. Excess glutamate leads to cell death and blocked transmission of signals across nerve synapses. Researchers are studying different drugs that may reduce glutamate binding among cells following spinal cord injury, which could reduce secondary cell death, improve motor function outcome, and reduce long-term hypersensitive pain postinjury.

REGENERATION

Neurons have a limited capacity to regenerate. As nerve cells are either damaged or destroyed by injury, and as others die naturally during development, the number of chemical interactions between adjacent nerve cells (synapses) decreases. Nerve cells can die when they do not make enough synapses, leaving large numbers of supporting glial cells in the area of damage. Glial cells are thought to support tissue after injury to the spinal cord but also inhibit the growth of axons.

Approaches to repairing damaged axons through remyelination and new growth include:

Some anti-inflammatory drugs have been shown to encourage axonal regeneration by stimulating CNS nerve axons to grow and by inhibiting amino acid toxicity and cell death that occurs after the initial injury. Two such nonsteroidal anti-inflammatory drugs are ibuprofen and indomethacin. The drug rolipram was shown to encourage axonal regeneration in an animal model of spinal cord injury. Preclinical studies are examining the effectiveness of rolipram in combination with other drugs given at different delivery times postinjury.

Antibodies are proteins made by immune cells and are designed to attach themselves to specific foreign proteins (called antigens) and disable them. Therapeutically, antibodies can be made that target specific proteins that inhibit repair of the body after injury. Monoclonal antibodies, produced in a laboratory, may promote nerve fiber regeneration by blocking proteins in the myelin debris that inhibit regeneration after spinal cord injury. Scientists are testing monoclonal antibodies at the site of the spinal cord injury in animal models in an attempt to block antiregeneration activity of cells in the damaged central nervous system and improve nerve function and recovery. For example, researchers are using a Nogo-A monoclonal antibody to block proteins that inhibit the sprouting and regeneration of axons following a spinal injury. Other antibodies, called anti-MAG (myelin associated glycoproteins), are designed to counteract protein-sugar molecules on myelin-forming debris at the site of injury.

A number of other targets are being tested to overcome inhibition to regeneration. Cethrin, a recombinant protein that blocks activation of rho (a protein that inhibits axon regeneration), has been tested clinically. A drug that targets Nogo-receptors is being developed to promote regeneration after spinal cord injury and stroke. Recent animal studies showing that inhibition of the tumor-suppressing gene PTEN can promote growth of upper motor neurons has led to active research into strategies to promote regeneration after spinal cord and optic nerve injuries. Finally, the histone deacetylases (HDAC) are a class of compounds that are involved in the regulation of gene expression and negatively affect cell structure following a traumatic spinal cord injury. Preclinical studies are examining ways to inhibit HDAC activity as a way to protect and allow axons to overcome inhibition in regions of a spinal injury.

To get past the glial scar that forms after a spinal cord injury and be able to transmit signals from the cell body, an axon has to advance between the tangles of long, branching molecules made up of inhibitory proteins and sugars that surround the cells. Experiments have successfully used a bacterial enzyme, chondroitinase ABC, to clear away the tangles so that axons could grow in animal models of injury. Researchers are looking at ways to combine chondroitinase ABC with other treatments, such as cell transplants, to increase functional recovery.

Other researchers are using a tissue-engineered highway-like matrix that is implanted onto the spinal cord to help axons "bridge" the lesion that forms at the injury site and to rebuild neural circuits. They also will look at using the matrix as a way of delivering growth factors that can promote nerve cell survival and inhibit proteins associated with the glial scar.

Cell Replacement

Controversy exists over potential benefits and possible harmful consequences of cell replacement and cell transplants. The potential of several cell types, including stem cells and glial cells, to treat spinal cord injury is being investigated eagerly, but there are many things about stem cells that researchers still need to understand. For example, researchers know there are many different kinds of chemical signals that tell a stem cell what to do. Some of these are internal to the stem cell, but many others are external—within the cellular environment—and will have to be recreated in the transplant region to encourage proper growth and differentiation. Because of the complexities involved in stem cell treatment, researchers expect these kinds of therapies to be possible only after some more researches are conducted. Preclinical research results are limited but show cell transplants can regenerate neuronal growth and create new connections between neurons.

Scientists are experimenting with a variety of cells for effectiveness and safety in increasing connectivity and restoring function following a spinal cord injury:

- Human oligodendrocyte progenitor cells have been shown to reduce secondary damage following a spinal cord injury and promote functional recovery and remyelination. Researchers are expanding trials to better determine optimal cell delivery windows and evaluate potential risks of transplants, such as the formation of tumors and inflammatory reactions
- Schwann cells surround and insulate peripheral nerves, and often grow into the spinal cord after injury. Schwann cells that have been transplanted at the site of the spinal cord injury can produce growth factors and reinsulate damaged nerve axons. They are not stem cells in that their fate as Schwann cells is determined before transplantation. Schwann cells can be taken from the individual's own body, which reduces the need for immune-suppressing drugs and the risk of tumor formation, but this requires several weeks after injury before grafting can be done. Preclinical studies are examining their potential in safely treating both acute and chronic spinal cord injury
- Bone marrow stromal cells, taken from the tissue found inside bones, have been shown in some studies to increase recovery from an injury to the spinal cord. Scientists are studying the injection of these cells into the cerebrospinal fluid (fluid that bathes the brain and spinal cord) to promote proteins needed to grow and maintain nerves and increase nerve signaling across the glial scarring that forms postinjury
- Nasal olfactory ensheathing cells, taken from the lining of the nose, are special types of glial cells that have been shown to promote axon regeneration and remyelination at the injury site. The transplanted cells have been shown to permit regrowth of axons in both the peripheral and central nervous systems, and improve functional outcome in animal models of spinal cord injury. Early-stage trials in humans are being conducted overseas.

Retraining CNS Circuits and Plasticity

Recovery from a spinal cord injury may occur for quite some time after the initial injury, as part of the brain's ability to reorganize or form new nerve connections and pathways following injury or cell death (called neuroplasticity).

Active Rehabilitation and Exercise

Specific training can improve function, coordination of fine muscle movements, and overall strength and health. Scientists are comparing the relative effectiveness of an intensive task-specific motor training program added to standard rehabilitation compared with standard rehabilitation alone for improving hand function and clinical outcomes in people with recent tetraplegia.

Epidural Stimulation

In May 2011, scientists funded in part by the National Institutes of Health reported that after intensive physical therapy and electrical stimulation to the spine, a man with a paralyzing spinal cord injury from the chest down had recovered the ability to stand and move paralyzed muscles at will when the stimulator is active. The man participated in a pilot study that combined epidermal stimulation and locomotor training—involving his being suspended for hours a day in a harness, walking on a treadmill while physical therapists moved his legs in stepping motions. Two years of locomotor training following his injury did not improve his ability to walk or stand. But he did improve after December 2009, when electrodes were surgically implanted over the paralyzed area of his spinal cord and began sending rhythmic electrical bursts to neurons in the spinal cord during the locomotor training sessions. This epidural simulation imitates the brain's sending signals to the spinal cord to begin movement. Gradually, he could became able to stand and fully bear his own weight for a few minutes at a time. Although he could not walk without assistance, he could bend one leg at the knee and flex his ankle when the stimulator is active. Locomotor training without any epidural stimulation is routinely used as a rehabilitative technique for people with spinal cord injuries—which allows some individuals to retain the ability to move and feel below the injury. Meanwhile, a form of epidural stimulation is used to relieve pain for some individuals. The researchers and NIH scientists caution that this finding was in only one person, and further study is required to confirm these early promising results and to understand exactly how the stimulation is working.

Functional Electric Stimulation

Exciting and promising results in restoring or assisting function in individuals with chronic spinal cord injury have been shown in studies using functional electric stimulation (FES). FES devices use a computer system and electrodes to deliver small bursts of a low-level electrical current to paralyzed muscles, to generate muscle contractions. Researchers are working to improve the electrode and computer interfaces so they can produce more natural yet complex movements. FES is being used to restore breathing without a ventilator, cough unassisted, enhance bladder and bowel control, increase hand movement and grasping, and improve blood flow to the skin.

Transcranial direct current stimulation (tDCS) is another form of electric stimulation that is being tested experimentally to improve patient outcomes after a spinal cord injury. tDCS is a noninvasive procedure that delivers continuous low electrical current to areas of the brain involved with movement via small electrodes placed on the scalp. Researchers are investigating if combining tDCS with exercise therapy for the affected hand will increase performance over exercise therapy alone. Other researchers hope to determine if tDCS can decrease chronic pain in people with spinal cord injury.

Robotic-assisted Therapy

Most recovery following SCI takes place within 6 months after injury. Substantial recovery after 12 months is unusual, but researchers continue to test ways to restore function in persons with chronic paralysis. In one very small study involving patients one year after injury, scientists are testing the safety and efficacy of a type of robotic therapy device known as the AMES device. The aim of this study is to investigate the use of assisted movement and enhanced sensation (AMES) technology in the rehabilitation of the legs of participants with incomplete spinal cord injury. The AMES device rotates the ankle over a range of 30 degrees while vibrators stimulate the tendons attached to muscles that move the leg. The subject's task is to assist the motion of the device.

In another study, researchers will determine the effect of using body-weight supported treadmill training and a robotic gait trainer on functional movement from place to place (ambulation) in people with an incomplete spinal cord injury. The person is suspended in a harness and onto a treadmill, and the robotic legs are strapped to the person. A computer controls the pace of the walking. The effect of the therapy will be evaluated by analyzing changes in ambulation and gait patterns during walking.

Brain–Computer Interfaces

The goal of brain-computer interface (BCI) technology is to bypass the damaged nerve circuits in the spinal cord and establish a direct link between the brain and an assistive implanted device which may restore an individual's control of voluntary muscle movement and coordination of paralyzed muscles.

Most individuals with tetraplegia have intact brain function but are unable to move due to injury or disease affecting the spinal cord. Brain-computer interface technology is based on the finding that with intact brain function, neural signals for movement are generated in the brain and can be used to control computer-assisted devices. By implanting electrodes in the brain, individuals can be trained to practice thoughts and thereby generate neural signals that are interpreted by a computer and translated to movement which can then be used to control a variety of devices or computer displays.

Researchers are working to develop BCI technology to offer individuals with upper limb paralysis a natural and rich control signal for prosthetic arms or FES device to reanimate paralyzed arms. The study uses electrocorticographic (ECoG) electrodes that interface with neurons in the brain's cortex (the part of the brain that is responsible for higher thought and motor control) to measure brain activity. Participants will learn to control computer cursors, virtual reality environments, and assistive devices, such as hand orthotics and FES devices using neural activity recorded with the ECoG sensor.

Another preliminary study is assessing the safety and effectiveness of a brain-computer interface to give people with tetraplegia the ability to control a computer cursor and other assistive devices with their thoughts. A small electrode array is inserted into the part of the brain's surface that controls movements. Using the very precise signals this device records, researchers are working to improve the computer's ability to interpret the person's intent and transfer that to the display screen.

4

Section

Recent Research
(SCI—Past, Present, Future)

Chapter Outline

37

Recent Research

Past: "An ailment not to be treated" and "They are destined to die" was the attitude and approach towards them from medical science (No Cure or No Care).

Present: After the world wars, Dr Munro and Dr Gutmann initiated the programs with medical/surgical/rehab care (Care but still No Cure).

Future: Many research projects are going on. Through technology, bridging the two ends of spinal cord is possible to transmit the impulses (cure and care).

- Stem cells are "undifferentiated" cells because they have not yet committed to developmental path that will form a specific tissue or organ. In some areas of our body, stem cells divide regularly to renew and repair the existing tissue. The bone marrow and gastrointestinal tract are examples of areas in which stem cells function to renew and repair tissue. The accessible sources of autologous adult cells in humans are:
  - Bone marrow—by drilling into bone and extracting (femur and iliac crest)
  - Adipose/lipid/fat cells—requires extraction by liposuction
  - Blood cells through "apheresis" wherein blood is drawn (like blood donation) and passed through a machine that extracts stem cells and returns blood.
- Pharmaceutic adjunct like Opiate blockers (naloxone), GM-1 ganglioside (Sysen), Thyrotropine releasing hormone (TRH), Erythropoietin
- Activated autologous macrophases.

- Bioengineering is continuously improving facilities for functions with technology. Bridging the injured ends of spinal cord with computer technology seems possible.
  - Schwann cells, olfactory ensheathing glial cells, matrix modifier with netrins and neural glues, peripheral micrograft
  - Regeneration/growth of axon shown promising results in animals with inhibitor neutralizing antibody
  - Replacing lost cells with stem cells and fetal tissue implants
  - Inhibit scar/gliosis formation
  - Reduce neurocircuit deficits with potassium and sodium channel blockers with glutamate receptor blockers.
- Robot rehabilitation: University of Zurich and Swiss Federal Institution have made study on spinal cord injured rat who could walk again with activation of innate intelligence and regenerative capacity
- Speech synthesizer: A California computer programmer developed a speaking program for Stephen Hawkins (a quadriplegic with aphasia) which is directed by head or eye ball movement. This allowed him to select words on computer screen that were then passed through a speech synthesizer to produce speech.

(All the research are not clear, consistent and without rewarding results).

38

Synthesis of Science with Spirituality

SCI rehabilitation requires objective treatment of medical, surgical and therapy and also subjective services of love, kind words, faith and motivation in the resettlement and rehabilitation process. Synthesis of Science with spirituality provides positivity to patient's psychology for a purpose in life and living. We have included two inspirational poems with the intention of encouraging patients and enhancing rehabilitation process.

"HOPE"

Climb up the rope of "Hope"
At every note, you will find a "scope",
Along with a message "don't stop"
Keep a watch with a "torch";
Get a "good coach" that can facilitate you,
To take you to the "Top"
Don't care whether you are,
Normal or abnormal, abled or disabled,
You do have a "Scope"
"Climb up! Climb up! Climb up!"

By Dinesh Sorani—the then B Physio student at Government Physio College, Ahmedabad. Now Sr. Lecturer at Physio College, Jamnagar

"DAWN"

Don't feel pity when you pass my side,
Once I was normal now on a blind ride.
In the midst of darkness, there came a "Guide"
Who said "fight" there is a ray of "light"
Who tried all the best to improve my "plight"
First I was bedridden, then on wheelchair,
Now I am walking, because of all the "care",
To face the world with my "dare".

By Sweta Patel—the then B Physio student, Government Physio College, Ahmedabad. At present as a Physio in USA.

39

Success Stories (Local): India

SHRI MUKUND RAI N PANDYA

Shri Pandya was born on 10th April, 1949 in a remote village Unchadi near Bhavnagar. Father died when he was 12. Illiterate mother worked as a water caress (giving drinking water at a railway station) and supported four children. After passing his 8th standard exam, in 1965 he developed Acute Transverse Myelitis, leaving behind paraplegia. He was admitted at Gondal hospital. After 7 days, he was transferred to Government Hospital, Bhavnagar. He was nearly on death bed when his emotional request to the then Health minister moved minister's heart and moved him to Government Civil Hospital, Ahmedabad after his 9 month's stay at Bhavnagar.

Medical rehabilitation: Here he received good medical and surgical care along with Rehab services of Physio-occupational therapy in B-1 Rehab Medicine Department at Civil Hospital, Ahmedabad. After sometime he realized that no more recovery is possible, he "accepted"

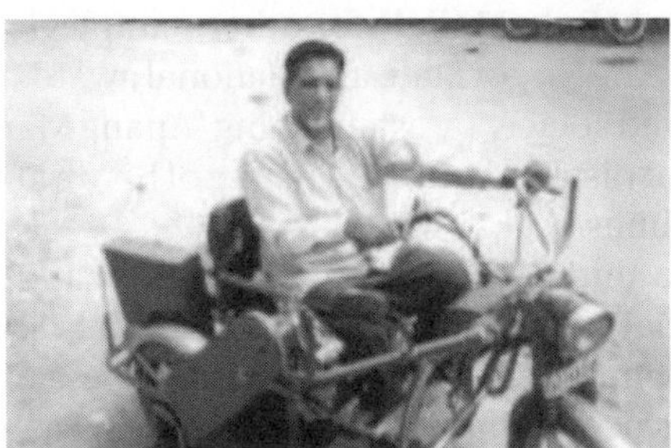

Fig. 1: A role model—Paraplegic Person, from Patient to PRO (Public Relation Officer). "A struggle for Existence—A struggle for Excellence", who lived a struggling but a successful and satisfying life with SCI for more than 45 years.

the disability and also the wheelchair life. He diverted his efforts toward rehab programs.

Educational rehabilitation: Now he thought and desired to continue studies. With the education minister's recommendations, without taking regular lectures in the school, he continued studies in the wards with the help of ward nurses and medical students along with his medical treatment and appeared to exams. He cleared his 11th standard exam on 7th trial which indicates his persistent persuasive struggle for studies inspite of his disability. He continued his studies and received Bachelor's degree and got his Journalism Diploma.

Vocational rehabilitation: He took primary training for telephone operator from the wards and typing practice in the Occupational therapy department B-1 at Civil Hospital, Ahmedabad. He got job as a telephone operator in civil hospital, still he was in the ward. He then took Government exam and got job as a Junior Clerk in Civil Hospital. With his educational qualification he got promoted as a medical social worker at Government Spine Hospital, Ahmedabad in 1985 and to the post of PRO in 1990, from where he retired from Government services in 2001.

Social rehabilitation: House and Home—He purchased his own house 8–9 km away from Civil Hospital and used motorized tricycle for transportation. During his job as Jr Clerk, he came in contact with Shobhana a totally abled girl and got married to her. She did good home making. Their children Shraddha and Arpit got good education and they got married with the help of their parents and got settled.

Excellence: Shri Pandya with wheelchair life served in Civil Hospital and in Government Spine Institute, Ahmedabad for nearly 25 years and become real "Role Model" for other paraplegic patients taking treatment. Shri Pandya got State and National awards and many other awards. He served society by establishing "Apang Manav Seva Sangh" for the welfare of disabled in 1979. Inspite of his disability he donated blood many a times.

Shri Pandya understood his medical, educational, vocational, family and social needs. Instead of just getting rehab services, he commanded, demanded from people and professionals and sought solutions for his needs. Shri Pandya got admitted as a patient in Civil Hospital and got retired as a PRO. He lived a fulfilling, satisfying, fully rehabilitated life as a paraplegic for more than 45 years and he died due to heart attack on 15 April, 2012 at the age of 63 years.

MADHVI RAMESHBHAI PANDYA

A quadriplegic who determined to do national flag hoisting in "Standing".

Madhavi then 14 years, lived happily with father, mother, three sisters and a brother in Amreli town. She is the youngest. Father had a small shop. She was studying in 8th grade. In life, sudden situations occur in such a way that what will happen is something that is inconceivable a moment before. Her elder sister had got engaged to a man. The annoyed youth rushed to Madhavi's home, with an intention to kill Madhvi's elder sister. Everyone from the house was away with some reason, except Madhavi. The angry youth argued with Madhavi and out of anger he assaulted her with a sharp weapon on her neck. A young girl, who was leading a joyful lively life, in fraction of seconds, was struggling for survival.

Madhvi was rushed to Amreli Hospital to Rajkot Hospital to Civil Hospital, Ahmedabad. After the primary care, she was transferred to Government Spine Hospital. She was given cervical traction with weights. Initially, there was no power in limbs, no sensation, no control over bladder and bowel. Nursing care prevented bed sore and urinary tract complications. Physiotherapy and occupational therapy in the wards improved the strength in the limbs. There was return of sensations. Afterwards she started attending Physiotherapy-Occupational therapy. With the progressive resistive exercises, the strength improved and then pregait training, then after gait training in the parallel bars to with walker to with a stick. With activities of daily living she became independent.

During her stay at the Institution, 56th Independence Day of India was celebrated. As a routing practice of the Institute, flag hoisting to be done by a SCI patient, she walked down to the flag pole and did flag hoisting. Patient and her parents were happy with the energetic and enthusiastic staff.

MRS PREMILABEN TEJABHAI AHIR

A paraplegic struggled to stand up to walk.

A victim of the most devastating and disastrous earthquake occurred with 7.5 Richter's scale with epicenter at Bhuj, which occurred on 26th January, 2001 in Kutchh district of Gujarat state of India, where lakhs where rendered homeless, 4–5 thousands were injured, 109 with spinal cord injury. The house of Premila where she dwelled turned into debris. She was lying underneath the debris in a semiconscious state for 2 days. On 3rd day she was rescued and shifted to Government Civil Hospital's intensive care unit (ICU), Ahmedabad. She was diagnosed L1 fracture with paralysis of both lower limbs with sensory loss and loss of control over bladder and bowel.

Operative management: Steffee fixation operation was performed.

Rehabilitation therapy: A spinal brace was given. She was given nursing, physio-occupational therapy. After few days, she was transferred to Government Spine Institute. She was allowed to sit gradually. From the wards, she came in wheelchair for the therapy. First she attended morning outdoor sports of OT dept. As there was return of muscle power in lower limbs, progressive resistive exercise and pregait training exercises were given in the Physio department. With bilateral posterior knee guards and bilateral toe raising splints, she was made to stand in the parallel bars and gait training was given, progressed to GT with walker to GT with a cane. In the OT department, she was trained for activities of daily living (ADL).

Social aspect: She belongs to a very poor family. She lived with father, mother and a younger brother. Premila was working as a laborer prior to the accident. Postinjury due to the disability her husband was reluctant to accept her. Effective counseling helped her to be with her husband.

Vocational rehabilitation: Medical social worker gave good counseling to bring her out of the trauma and the social and vocational issues. Because of disability, she could not go back to her work as a laborer. She was encouraged to continue and improve traditional world famous Kuchhi embroidery and knitting work. A sewing machine was donated to her on discharge.

Sports: On the previous day of Independence Day, on 14th August, sports competition was organized by OT department, she participated and won the first prize in the shot put game.

Event celebrations: She performed the Flag hoisting on the Independence Day in the campus.

Premila is living happily and independently with her husband. She is earning her bread and butter by embroidery and tailoring. She is also gets Rs. 2000/month as a pension from Government of Gujarat.

MRS AMINABEN

Earthquake affected paraplegic running a beauty parlor.

Aminaben was living and leading a happy and healthy life with her husband and two sons in the city of Bhuj-Kutchh, Gujarat. The earthquake on 26th January, 2001 shattered her total life. House became debris, lost her one son, she was buried under debris and became paraplegic, and husband was not cooperating well. From this grave situation her journey started for recovery and rehabilitation. She was taken to Bidada Sarvoday Trust Hospital 60 km away from Bhuj. Here she was operated upon and therapeutic measures were started. Along with the problems of house, husband, paralysis and the grief of losing her son continued lingering and bothering her.

During her stay at Bidada hospital, the Safari from Government Spine Hospital, Ahmedabad, visited the hospital where 20 SCI and 300 other patients were being treated. The team advised her to get transferred to Ahmedabad.

Therapy: At Government Spine Institute, a regular rehabilitation program started. She was given psychological counseling, and started attending Physio-Occupational therapy. The scientifically designed therapeutic exercises gave her gradual improvement and finally she started walking with a deviated gait. She had sensory recovery also. She became independent in her ADL as well.

Vocation: After her stay of three months, she was discharged. Medical social work department studied her socioeconomic status and advised

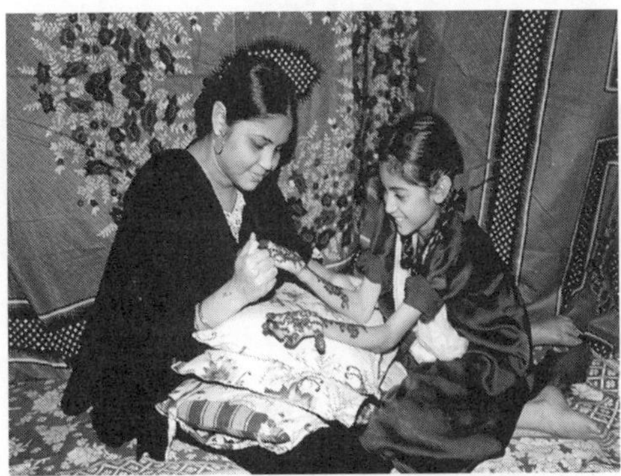

Fig. 2: Mrs Aminaben

her for beauty parlor saloon for vocational rehabilitation. On discharge she went to her father's home.

Second set back: She was trying her level best to settle in a new life style. Another aftershock of earthquake shattered her program, her husband left her. She started staying in a relief camp, where the Safari team on their follow-up program met her. The team contacted NGO of Bhuj to arrange a training program of Beauty parlor course; they readily arranged it and gave assurance to help her in all possible way. Again she started struggling to settle down confidently.

Meanwhile, Govt of Gujarat declared pension scheme for all earthquake affected SCI patients. She started getting Rs. 2000/month as a pension. Government also provided a new house to her. After hearing all these benefits, her husband returned to her. With these help—house husband, pension, beauty parlor, she is out of the tragedy and now living happy life.

MR RAJESH KHUMANSINH RATHOD

Rajesh—A painter with paraplegia.

A resident of village Killa Pardi near Valsad district, Gujarat. One day he went to a nearby village in-spite of his parent's denial. On returning, he took a ride on his friend's bike. When they were about to reach home, his friend lost his control over the bike and they met with an accident. His friend was drunk and he died on the spot. The accident gave him fracture of the spine and paralysis of both lower limbs.

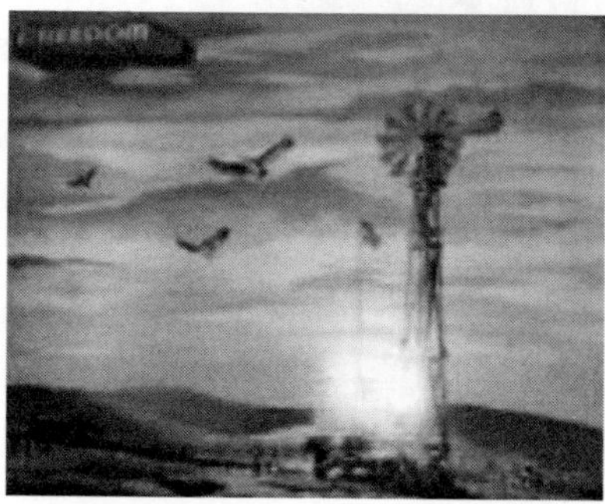

Fig. 3: "FREEDOM" message

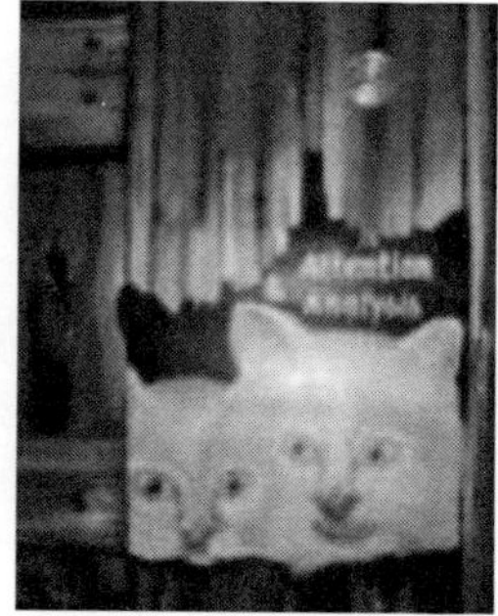

Fig. 4: Attention and analysis

He was admitted in the Government Spine Institute. With the help of therapy program, he became independent with wheelchair and in ADL. He got good guidance as regards to changes in the bathroom, toilet and kitchen to remove architectural barriers.

He thoughtfully compared Rehab program with the exam papers.

a. First paper: Mental—To overcome depression and put mind on the track of Rehab process is a very hard paper. Once you conquer your depression, 90% of your disability is gone.
b. Second paper: Physical—He thanked the PT and OT department for exercises of upper, lower limbs and trunk and teaching how to transfer from bed to wheelchair and back. All the exercises made him mobile and the second paper became easy for him.
c. Third Paper: Economy—It is successfully cleared by learning the vocation of one's aptitude like music, sewing, painting, embroidery, computer, etc. by which a person can earn money. Also the person's brain is engaged so that depressive thoughts do not trouble him or her.
d. Fourth paper: Social—The last paper can be cleared by the love, affection and the necessary help from the family and friends. Mr Rajesh was a good painter. He painted many memorable paintings with oil paints during his stay in the hospital. All the paintings had some meaningful message. He continued this work at home after discharge and earned Rs.12000-15000/month. He gave good advice to all "Never ever disobey your parent, elder and Guru's advice". He thinks that he met with an accident and became paralyzed because he didn't obey his parent's advice of not going to nearby village.

MRS BHAVNA RAJESH PADIA

(A doctor's wife with paraplegia gained walking.)

Dr Rajesh Padia, as well known plastic surgeon of Maninagar area of Ahmedabad was living happily with his wife Bhavna (35), one son and a daughter. On 26th January, 2001 earthquake came and gone, destroying the life of Dr. Rajesh's family. Dr. Rajesh and his 5 years old son died in their house which collapsed and Bhavna and her daughter buried in the debris who were rescued after 28 hours. The family and the friend circle were having a very good educational and financial background. They admitted her in a private hospital. Bhavna suffered a spinal cord injury with paraplegia. Daughter had minor injuries.

Bhavna was operated for her spine injury. She stayed there for one month time. She got physiotherapy there. One relative advised them to transfer her to Government Spine Institute.

The grief of losing her husband and son and also the fear of lifelong bedridden position, lost her interest in life. Situation made her depressed and melancholy. This problem created a hindrance in her active participation in the rehab program. But the ability and the knack of the rehab team to tackle such patients tactfully harnessed her energy for her active participation.

Rehab services—She attended physio-occupational therapy. The exercises helped her muscles to regain strength and stamina. Stage by stage, she finally started standing in the parallel bars with posterior knee guard and toe raising splints for dropped feet. She showed good progress reaching to a stage of walking with a cane. She also became self-sufficient in her day-to-day activities.

On discharge, at one time a totally depressed Bhavna, became independent in her life. She complimented the hospital by comparing it with a "Manav Mandir Hospital—a temple of humanity."

40

Success Stories (Global): International Personalities

Dr TED RUMMEL

Paraplegic orthopedic doing Surgeries—Missouri.

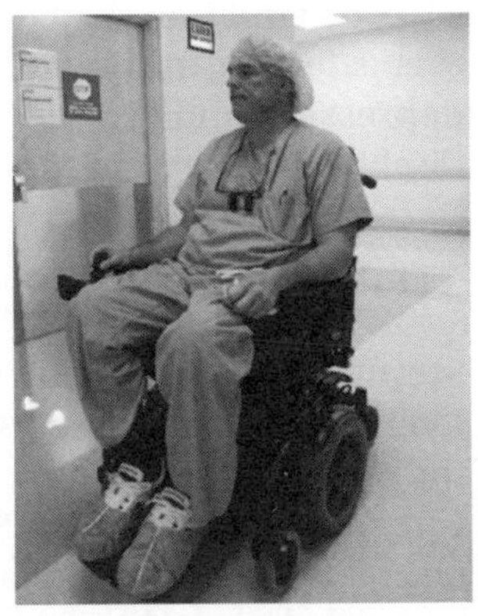

Fig. 1: Dr Ted Rummel

Dr Rummel lost his ability to stand and walk when a blood-filled cyst on his spine burst in 2010 with the paralysis from waist down. A year of intense rehabilitation, family and friend's sustained support, and with an ingenious stand up wheelchair, he is back in game at work seeing patients and performing knee, foot, ankle and elbow surgeries.

Now the tenacious orthopedic surgeon can do virtually everything of his own which he could do previously.

He maintains his physical strength with exercises and mental and emotional strength with deeply devoted work of patient's care.

FRANKLIN D ROOSEVELT

President Franklin D Roosevelt was born on 30th January, 1882 in New York. He got married to Anna Eleanor in 1905 and they had 6 children. In 1921, while vacationing in Canada, Roosevelt contracted Polio, which resulted in permanent paralysis from the waist down for the rest of his life. He tried a wide range of therapies, including Hydrotherapy. In 1926, he purchased a resort at Warm spring, Georgia, where he founded a hydrotherapy center for the treatment of the polio patients, one which still operates.

Fitting his hips and legs with iron braces, he laboriously taught himself to walk a short distance by swiveling his torso while supporting himself with two canes; otherwise he used wheelchair for mobility.

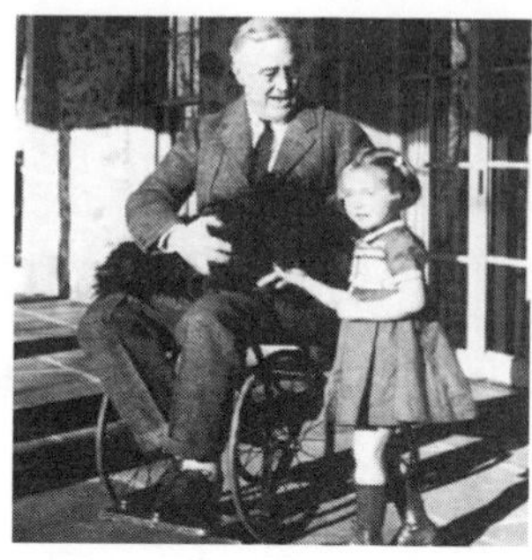

Fig. 2: US president with polio paraplegia

He was the 32nd President of US. He served as a President for three terms, from March 4, 1933 to April 12, 1945 till he died, the only president who was in the office for more than 8 years. In spite of his paralysis problem and disability, he worked as a powerful President of US. He was the central figure in the world events, leading the United States during a time of worldwide economic depression and World War II. He proved that "Impairment and disability need not become a handicap."

STEPHEN HAWKING

Stephen Hawking was born on 8th January, 1942 in Oxford, UK. In 1963, at the age of 21, Hawking was diagnosed with Amyotrophic Lateral Sclerosis (ALS or Lou Gehrig's disease) and was given 2 years to live, yet he went to Cambridge to become a brilliant researcher and professorial fellow at Gonville College.

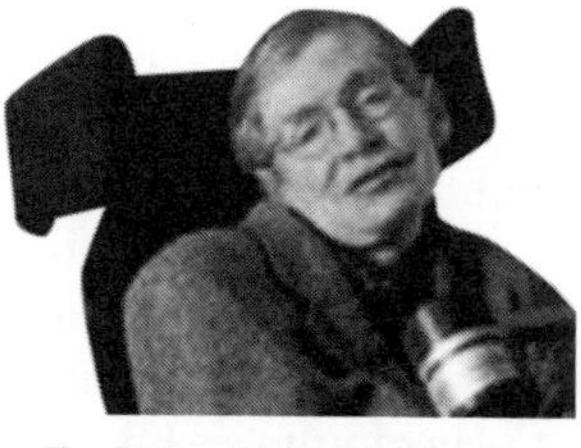

Fig. 3: A noted scientist with quadriplegia

Professor earned his PhD and has a dozen of honorary degrees and many awards. In 1965, he married to Jane Wilde, got divorced in 1995. Married second time to Elaine Mason in 1995 and got divorced in 2006. He has three children.

Despite his debilitating illness, he has done ground-breaking work in physics and cosmology, and his several books have helped to make science accessible to everyone. In a sense, Hawking's disease helped him become the noted scientist, he is today. Before the diagnosis, Hawking hadn't always focused on his studies. With sudden realization that he might not even live long enough to earn his PhD, he focused on studies.

Withphysical control over his body diminished, he was forced to use a wheelchair. In mid 1970s, Hawking's family had taken in one of Hawking's graduate students to help manage his care and work. He could still feed himself and get out of bed, but virtually for everything else, he required assistance. In addition, his speech had become increasingly slurred. In 1985, he lost his voice for good, following a tracheostomy. The resulting situation required 24-hour nursing care; for the acclaimed physicist. A California computer programmer developed a speaking program that could be directed by head or eyeball movement. This allowed him to select words on a computer screen that were then passed through a speech synthesizer. Today, with virtually all control of his body gone, Hawking directs wheelchair through a cheek muscle attached to a sensor.

CHRISTOPHER REEVE

A superman of film with quadriplegia.

Christopher Reeve was born on 25 September, 1952, in New York USA, was an American actor, film director, producer, screen writer, author and activist. He achieved stardom for his acting achievements, in particular his motion-picture portrayed of the DC comic book superhero, Superman.

Reeve married to Dana Morosini in April 1992. On 27 May, 1995, Reeve became quadriplegic after being thrown from a horse during an equestrian competition in Virginia. He required a wheelchair and breathing apparatus for the rest of his life. Reeve became the face of spinal cord injury and inspired a new generation of Medical and Rehab scientists to focus on recovery and improving quality of life for SCI. Ideas from gene therapy to stem cell transplantation and a new outlook on Rehab with psycho, socio, vocational along with physical mobility gave a boost to a better remaining life of SCI. Christopher and Dana Reeve foundation for Paralysis Resource Center is established, serving the needs of people with disabilities.

Multiple Choice Questions (MCQs)

1. The shock that follows an injury to thoracolumbar segment of spinal cord is caused by:
   a. Vasodilatation
   b. Heart failure
   c. Blood loss
   d. Sudden epinephrine release.
2. At what point is it permissible to release manual in line immobilization of Head and Neck?
   a. Once the patient understands that he should not move the head
   b. Once a cervical collar is applied
   c. Once the patient's head is secured to a long spine board
   d. Once the patient is positioned (unsecured) on a long spine board.
3. Which statement concerning spinal cord injury is not true?
   a. Anterior cord syndrome is caused by the compression of the artery supplying anterior spinal cord
   b. Brown sequard's syndrome can be caused by the bullet that completely transects the spinal cord
   c. Central cord syndrome could be caused by the hyperextension of the cervical spine
   d. Posterior cord syndrome is caused by the compression of the posterior spinal artery.
4. A patient who suffered a complete transaction of the cord at T4 level will exhibit which of the following:
   a. The patient will not have sensation below the nipple line
   b. The patient will not be able to move the upper extremities

   c. The patient will not have sensation from the shoulders down
   d. The patient will not have sensation around and below the umbilicus.
5. Which of the following describes central cord lesion?
   a. Central cord syndrome typically shows weakness of upper extremities
   b. Central cord syndrome has high prognosis for recovery
   c. Central cord syndrome is often associated with preexisting degenerative disease
   d. All of the above are true.
6. Which of the following drug should be considered in SCI, not responding to fluid challenge?
   a. Dexamethazone
   b. Methyl prednisone
   c. Decadron
   d. Dopamine.
7. When immobilizing the head of a young child, it may be necessary to:
   a. To pad behind the child's shoulders
   b. To pad behind the child's head, neck, shoulders
   c. To pad behind the child's head
   d. To pad behind the child's head and shoulders.
8. Which of the following mechanism suggests a cervical spine injury?
   a. Gunshot wound to head
   b. Patient involved in a rear end impact motor vehicle collision
   c. Sledding accident in which patient thrown down a hill
   d. All of the above.
9. Which of the following signs will not be associated with a spinal cord injury?
   a. Priapism
   b. Positive Babinski's response
   c. Right-sided facial paralysis
   d. Hands up positioning.
10. The cervical spine accounts for:
    a. Less than 10% of all spinal cord injury
    b. Less than 50% of all spinal cord injury
    c. More than 25% of all spinal cord injury
    d. More than 50% of all spinal cord injury.

11. Which of these facts about spinal cord is correct?
    a. There are 30 pairs of nerves that exit the cord
    b. The spinal cord extends down to the level of 5th lumbar vertebra
    c. The spinal cord is anchored to the coccyx by filum terminale
    d. Gray matter is superficial to the white matter of the spinal cord.
12. The most superficial of the meninges is the:
    a. Arachnoid matter
    b. Pia matter
    c. Dura matter
    d. Conus medullaris.
13. In a cross-section of the spinal cord, the peripheral white portion consists of___ forming nerve tracts and the central gray portion consists of____
    a. Dendrites, axon
    b. Unmyelinated axons, neuron cell bodies
    c. Myelinated axons, sensory receptors
    d. Myelinated axons, neuron cell bodies.
14. The anterior (ventral) horn of the spinal cord contains the cell bodies of
    a. Motor neurons to skeletal muscles
    b. Sensory neurons
    c. Associated neurons
    d. To the funiculous.
15. The spinal nerves
    a. Contains sensory axons
    b. Contains motor axons
    c. Are formed from the convergence of dorsal and ventral roots
    d. Exit the ventral column via the intervertebral foramina
    e. All of the above.
16. Given these components of a reflex: 1. Association neuron; 2. Skeletal muscle; 3. Afferent neuron: 4. Efferent neuron; 5. Sensory receptors. Choose the sequence below that best represents the order followed in a reflex from stimulus to response.
    a. 5 4 3 2 1
    b. 5 3 2 4 1
    c. 5 4 3 1 2
    d. 5 3 1 4 2

17. Reflexes
    a. Are never homeostatic
    b. Are automatic responses to a stimulus
    c. Can't be suppressed by higher brain functions
    d. Are always simple pathways containing three neurons.
18. Stretch reflex
    a. Cause muscle to contract in response to a stretching force applied to them
    b. Involve a sensory receptor (muscle spindle)
    c. Involves sensory neuron that directly synapses with motor neurons in spinal cord
    d. Help maintain posture
    e. All of the above.
19. A knee jerk reflex is an example of
    a. Cross extensor reflex
    b. Withdrawal reflex
    c. Golgi tendon reflex
    d. Stretch reflex.
20. The Golgi tendon reflex
    a. Involves the synapse of sensory neurons from the Golgi tendon organs with stimulating interneurons at the spinal cord
    b. Prevents contracting muscles from applying excessive tension to tendons
    c. Involves the stimulation of alpha neurons leading back to muscles that are stretching tendons
    d. Results in increased tension at tendons.
21. The withdrawal reflex
    a. Includes the Golgi tendon organ
    b. Includes the synapse of sensory neurons directly with alpha neurons
    c. Helps to protects body from painful stimuli
    d. Is a response to increased tension at tendon.
22. Which of these events occur when a person step a tack with right foot?
    a. The right foot is pulled away from the tack because of golgi tendon reflex (GTR)
    b. The left leg is extended to support the body because of stretch reflex

c. The flexors of thigh contract and extensors relax because of reciprocal innervation
d. The extensors of both thighs contract because of the crossed extensor reflex.

23. Dorsal rami of spinal nerve innervates
    a. Anterior neck muscles
    b. Deep back muscles
    c. Intercostal muscles
    d. Muscles of upper limbs.
24. Which is the most common site of spinal cord injury?
    a. Thoracolumbar segment
    b. Lower cervical spine
    c. Upper cervical spine
    d. Sacral spine.
25. All of the following are true about spinal injuries except
    a. About 80% of spinal injuries result in neurological deficit
    b. Thoracolumbar spine injury may result in paraplegia
    c. Cervical spine injury may result in quadriplegia
    d. Any lesion to the spinal cord above T5 causes hypotension.
26. The nucleus pulposus is a remnant of
    a. Sclerotomes
    b. Occipital myotome
    c. Notochord
    d. Mesenchyme.
27. The entire vertebral column has similar articulation except
    a. C1–C2
    b. C7–T1
    c. T12–L1
    d. L5–S1.
28. The adjacent laminae of the vertebrae are joined together by
    a. Ligamentum teres
    b. Ligamentum flavum
    c. Ligament of treitz
    d. Anterior longitudinal ligament.
29. *Assertion:* Pure dislocation (without associated fracture) doesn't occur in the lumbar spine. *Reason:* The facets of the lumbar spine are stout and vertically placed whereas cervical spine facets are short and more horizontally placed.
    a. Assertion is true but reasoning is false
    b. Assertion is false but reasoning is true

c. Both are true
d. Both are false.

30. ASH brace is used for
    a. Dorsolumbar spine injury
    b. Cevical spine injury
    c. Both
    d. None.
31. SOMI brace is used for
    a. Thoracic spine injury
    b. Cervical spine injury
    c. Lumbar spine injury
    d. All.
32. Clay shoveller's fracture is a fracture of the spinous process of which vertebra.
    a. C1
    b. T1
    c. L1
    d. C2.
33. What is the name of the skull calipers used for skull traction for the reduction of cervical spine fracture?
    a. Crutchfield tongs traction
    b. Hutchinson's tong traction
    c. Trendelenburg tong traction
    d. Gopalan's tong traction.
34. In which type of injury traction doesn't help?
    a. Vertical compression injury
    b. Extension injury
    c. Direct injury
    d. Flexion rotation injury.
35. All of the following regarding the diagnosis of spinal injuries are true except
    a. A tomogram helps in better delineation of a doubtful area
    b. Myelogram has proved to be a very helpful investigation in acute spinal injuries
    c. One can see damaged structures more clearly with CT scan
    d. MRI is the best modality of imaging in an injured spine.
36. In which of the following types of spinal injury, the plain X-ray appears normal in the presence of highly unstable spinal injury?
    a. Fall from height on buttocks
    b. Strong hit on the shoulders

c. Whiplash injury to the cervical spine
d. Bullet injury to the spine.

37. Which of the following type of spinal injury occurs due to seat belt while driving
    a. Flexion injury
    b. Flexion-rotation injury
    c. Extension injury
    d. Flexion-distraction injury.
38. Which of the following is commonly associated with burst fracture of spine?
    a. Flexion injury
    b. Flexion-rotation injury
    c. Vertical compression injury
    d. Extension injury.
39. The neural arches of adjacent vertebrae articulate through which joint.
    a. Ball and socket joint
    b. Facet joints
    c. Both
    d. None.
40. A 56-year-old female with a diagnosis of a herniated disc between C6–C7. During a conversation with physician, he informs you that the patient has a C7 nerve root impingement. Upon testing this patient, you expect weakness in all of the following motor activities except for which one.
    a. Wrist flexion
    b. Finger flexion
    c. Finger extension
    d. Elbow extension.
41. You are teaching a spinal cord injury patient, proper pressure relief in the wheelchair. You explain that every 10–15 minutes he will need to provide pressure relief-independent to prevent sores. What is the minimal level of injury this patient can have, in order to be able to provide independent care for himself?
    a. C4
    b. C5
    c. C6
    d. C8.
42. You are instructed to perform manual muscle testing on a L3–L4 SCI patient, who is a 21-year-old male and uncooperative. Which of the following considerations is not important?

a. Informing the patient of what you will be doing
b. Stabilizing the patient's proximal part
c. Lining up the origin and insertion
d. Testing bilaterally, starting with the injuries side first.

43. The patient is sent to you for bracing as a result of a fracture at the level T10 to L1. The physician recommends a rigid high back brace for stabilization. Which of the following braces would be most appropriate to plan for this patient?
    a. Lumbar corset
    b. Taylor brace
    c. Knight-Taylor spinal brace
    d. Jewett brace.
44. During your physical therapy studies, you are learning about Spina bifida disorders. Which of the following describes Spina bifida myelomeningocele?
    a. A soft tissue tumor in the meninges
    b. A soft tissue tumor in the spinal cord
    c. The most severe form of Spina bifida
    d. A herniated sac within the spinal cord.
45. A patient reports to physical therapy with a diagnosis of a lesion in the lateral cord of the brachial plexus. Which of the following would you most likely to detect upon evaluation of this patient?
    a. Paralysis of biceps, coracobrachialis and finger flexors
    b. Paralysis of deltoid
    c. Paralysis of wrist extension
    d. Paralysis of hand intrinsic.
46. A patient was diagnosed of herniated disc at the L4. Which of the following will have the most weakness?
    a. Knee flexion
    b. Ankle dorsi flexion
    c. Knee extension
    d. Hip flexion.
47. A patient with spinal accessory nerve injury will have difficulty in
    a. Shrugging the shoulder
    b. Adduction of scapula
    c. External rotation of shoulder
    d. Horizontal adduction of shoulder.
48. A PT is assigned to do discharge plan for a SCI patient. The therapist's first step would be

a. Home assessment report from PT/OT/MSW prior to discharge
b. Make a visit to patient's house when you find time
c. Get information from patient's relatives
d. No need about the house information.

49. A PT is evaluating a patient with acute lumbar disc protrusion. "Least" indicator to discharge the patient is
a. The pain problem is decreased as per the goals set in treatment plan
b. The patient understands the back care
c. Repeated backward bending centralizes the pain
d. The pain problem is increased as per the goals set in the treatment plan.

50. Bulbocavernosus reflex indicates
a. It indicates presence of complete spinal cord injury
b. Termination of the spinal shock
c. Positive anal sphincter contraction
d. All of the above
e. None of the above.

ANSWERS

1. a. Vasodilation: The sympathetic nervous system exits the spinal cord from thoracolumbar segment. After injury sympathetic system is compromised and parasympathetic system dominates causing vasodilation and shock.
2. c. Once the patient's head is secured to a long spine board, this will effectively prevent patient from moving head and neck.
3. b. Brown...occurs when there is partial injury with ipsilateral signs and symptoms.
4. a. T4 cord lesion has sensory loss and paralysis below nipple line.
5. d. All are true. Upper limbs are more affected; prognosis is better and is associated with degeneration.
6. d. Dopamine. The continuous use of steroid such as Dexamethazone, Methyl prednisone, Decadron is no longer recommended.
7. a. Behind shoulder...Young children have large occipital region that can cause head and neck flexion. It may be prudent to place a bulky pad underneath the shoulder to maintain neutral in line position.

8. d. All the above mechanism of injury can cause cervical spine injury.
9. c. Spinal column does not influence the muscles of face in an isolated cord injury.
10. d. The cervical spine represents a segment of the spinal column where the cord is largest and the spinal cavity is smallest. Additionally, the mobile head places the neck and cervical spine in a precipitous position for a cervical cord injury.
11. c. The spinal cord is anchored to the coccyx by filum terminale.
12. c. Dura mater. Conus medullaris is not meninges. It is the cone like inferior end of the spinal cord.
13. d. White portion—myelinated axons, Gray portion—Neuron cell bodies.
14. a. Motor neurons to skeletal muscles.
15. e. All the above.
16. d. 5. Sensory receptors 3. Afferent neuron 1. Association neuron 4. Efferent neuron 2. Skeletal muscle.
17. b. Are automatic responses to a stimulus, reflexes are homeostatic.
18. e. All of above.
19. d. Muscle is stimulated to contract in response to a stretch reflex.
20. b. Prevents contracting muscles from applying excessive tension to tendon.
21. c. Helps to protect body from painful stimuli. GTO is not a withdrawal reflex.
22. c. The thigh flexors contracts and extensors relax due to reciprocal innervation.
23. b. Deep back muscles.
24. a. Thoracolumbar segment.
25. a. About 20% of spinal injuries result in neurological deficit.
26. c. Notochord.
27. a. C1–C2.
28. b. Ligamentum flavum.
29. c. Both are true.
30. a. ASH—Anterior Spinal Hyperextension brace for Dorsolumbar spine injury.
31. b. SOMI—Sterno-occipital Mandibular Immobilization for cervical spine injury.
32. b. T1.
33. a. Crutchfield tongs traction
34. b. Extension injury caused by vehicular accident and shallow water diving leading to avulsion fracture of anterior lip of vertebra

C5–C6 and lumbar spine, most commonly involved. There is only anterior column failure, a stable fracture.

35. b. Myelogram is not useful in an acute injury.
36. c. In whiplash injury to the cervical spine, all three columns of the spine are disrupted in a sudden hyperflexion followed by sudden hyperextension of the neck. Sudden stopping of a car, sudden jerk on leg while walking with heavy weight on head.
37. d. Flexion-distraction injury.
38. c. Vertical compression fracture.
39. b. Facet joint.
40. b. Finger flexion.
41. c. C6 Independent care of himself; At C4, patient is able only to direct pressure relief activities; At C5, patient is Independent in pressure relief; At C8, patient is independent in pressure including, wheelchair and push ups.
42. d. Testing, starting with noninjured side first, then comparing to injured side.
43. c. Knight Taylor brace is for fracture above L3. Lumbar corset is soft and is not for fracture. Taylor brace is semirigid and used for thoracic and lumbar diseases (not fractures). Jewett brace is a three point brace that prevents hyperextension.
44. c. Myelomeningocele—spinal canal remain open at several vertebrae, protective membrane (meninges) and spinal cord protrusion, is the most severe form. Meningocele-meninges protrude out. Syringomyelocele—a herniated sac in spinal cord. Occulta (mildest-no disability)—defective closure of lamina without spinal cord or meninges protrusion (lumbosacral region with tuft of hair).
45. a. Paralysis of biceps, coracobrachialis, finger flexors. Deltoid paralysis is due to axillary nerve lesion. Paralysis of intrinsics of hand is due to medial cord lesion. Paralysis of wrist extensors is due to posterior cord lesion.
46. b. Ankle dorsiflexion.
47. a. Shrugging of scapula.
48. a. Home assessment report by PT/OT/MSW prior to the discharge.
49. c. Patient understands the back care is the most indicator. This option is a diagnostic criterion whereas the other three can have an influence in discharge decision. a. and b. are taken into consideration during discharge.
50. d. All of the above.

Information of Some Spinal Cord Injury Centers

NATIONAL (INDIAN) SPINAL CORD INJURY CENTERS

1. Government Spine Institute—Civil Hospital Ahmedabad, Gujarat 380016.
2. Government Spine ward—SSG Hospital, Vadodara, Gujarat.
3. Indian Spinal Injury Center, Sector-C, Vasant kunj, New Delhi-110070.
4. Orthopedic N Spine Center—Pal hospital. Jalandhar city, Punjab 144001.
5. Apollo Hospital, Asha Rehab Center. Chennai, Tamilnadu.
6. Armed forces—Paraplegia Rehab unit. Kirki, near Pune, Maharastra.
7. All India Institute of Rehab center. Hajiali, Mumbai, Maharashtra.
8. Christian Medical College, CMC, Vellore, Tamil Nadu.
9. Regional Spinal Injury Center. Cuttack, Odhissa.
10. Sharan Spinal Rehab Center. Mumbai, Maharashtra.
11. Spinal Rehab Center. Amritsar, Punjab.
12. Spinal Injury Center. Safdarjung Hospital, New Delhi.
13. Nina foundation, One World Spinal Rehab Center. Bombay, Maharastra.
14. Hope Rehab Center, Patna, Bihar.

INTERNATIONAL SPINAL CORD INJURY CENTERS

1. Christopher and Dana Reeve foundation. New Jersey, USA.
2. Gutmann's Stoke Mandeville National Spinal Injury Center. Aylesbury Bucks, UK.

3. Kennedy Krieger Institute. Baltimore, USA.
4. Magee-Regional Spinal Cord Injury Center. Philaldelphia, USA.
5. Heidelberg University Hospital's Spinal Cord Injury Center. Heildelberg, Germany.
6. National Spinal Cord Injury Association. New York, USA.
7. Santa Clara Valley Medical Center for Rehabilitation. California, USA.
8. Regional Spinal Cord Injury Care of Southern California USA.
9. Munroe Regional Medical Center Florida USA.
10. Royal Ottawa Rehabilitation Center for Spinal Cord Injury. Canada.
11. Toronto Spinal Cord Injury Rehab Center. Canada.
12. Mooring spinal unit, Royal Rehabilitation Center. Sydney, Australia.
13. Center for Rehabilitation of Paralyzed, Sarvar Dhaka Bangladesh.
14. Copenhagen University hospital: Clinic for para and tetraplegia. Hornbaek, Denmark.
15. National Institute of Medical Rehabilitation. Budapest, Hungary.

Bibliography

BOOKS AND ARTICLES ON SPINAL CORD INJURY

1. Across the street from hell: My Spinal Cord Injury Recovery. By Mark Anthony Hall.
2. A Manual on Sexuality for Men with Spinal Cord Injury. By Robert W. Baer.
3. Baskin DS. Spinal cord injury. New York: Oxford University Press. 2006.
4. Beattie MS, et al. Endogenous repair after spinal cord contusion injuries in the rat. Experimental neurology. 1997;148(2):453-63.
5. Behrman AL, Harkema SJ. Locomotor training after human spinal cord injury: a series of case studies. Physical Therapy. 2000;80(7):688-700.
6. Bethea JR, et al. Traumatic spinal cord injury induces nuclear factor-κB activation. The Journal of neuroscience. 1998;18(9):3251-60.
7. Blight AR, Decrescito V. Morphometric analysis of experimental spinal cord injury in the cat: the relation of injury intensity to survival of myelinated axons. Neuroscience. 1986;19(1):321-41.
8. Blight AR. Cellular morphology of chronic spinal cord injury in the cat: analysis of myelinated axons by line-sampling. Neuroscience. 1983;10(2):521-43.
9. Blight AR. Macrophages and inflammatory damage in spinal cord injury. Journal of neurotrauma. 1992;9:S83-91.
10. Bracken MB, et al. Administration of methylprednisolone for 24 or 48 hours or tirilazad mesylate for 48 hours in the treatment of acute spinal cord injury: results of the Third National

Acute Spinal Cord Injury Randomized Controlled Trial. Jama. 1997;277(20):1597-604.

11. Bracken MB, et al. A randomized, controlled trial of methylprednisolone or naloxone in the treatment of acute spinal-cord injury: results of the Second National Acute Spinal Cord Injury Study. New England Journal of Medicine. 1990;322(20):1405-11.
12. Bracken MB, et al. Efficacy of methylprednisolone in acute spinal cord injury. Jama. 1984;251(1):45-52.
13. Bracken MB, et al. Methylprednisolone or naloxone treatment after acute spinal cord injury: 1-year follow-up data: results of the second National Acute Spinal Cord Injury Study. Journal of neurosurgery. 1992;76(1):23-31.
14. Bracken MB, et al. Methylprednisolone or tirilazad mesylate administration after acute spinal cord injury: 1-year follow-up: Results of the third National Acute Spinal Cord Injury randomized controlled trial. Journal of neurosurgery. 1998;89(5):699-706.
15. Bradbury EJ, et al. Chondroitinase ABC promotes functional recovery after spinal cord injury. Nature. 2002;416(6881):636-40.
16. Bregman BS, et al. Neurotrophic factors increase axonal growth after spinal cord injury and transplantation in the adult rat. Experimental neurology. 1997;148(2):475-94.
17. Bregman BS, et al. Recovery from spinal cord injury mediated by antibodies to neurite growth inhibitors. 1995;498-501.
18. Bryce TN. Spinal Cord Injury. Demos Medical Publishing. 2009.
19. Bunge RP, et al. Observations on the pathology of human spinal cord injury. A review and classification of 22 new cases with details from a case of chronic cord compression with extensive focal demyelination. Advances in neurology. 1993;59:75.
20. Carlson SL, et al. Acute inflammatory response in spinal cord following impact injury. Experimental neurology. 1998;151(1): 77-88.
21. Chopp M, et al. Spinal cord injury in rat: treatment with bone marrow stromal cell transplantation. Neuroreport. 2000;11(13):3001-5.
22. Crewe NM, Krause JS. "Spinal Cord Injury." Medical, Psychosocial and Vocational Aspects of Disability. 1979;289.
23. Crowe MJ, et al. Apoptosis and delayed degeneration after spinal cord injury in rats and monkeys. Nature Medicine. 1997;3(1): 73-6.

24. De Groat WC, et al. Mechanisms underlying the recovery of urinary bladder function following spinal cord injury. Journal of the autonomic nervous system. 1990;30:S71-S77.
25. DeVivo MJ, Black KJ, Stover SL. Causes of death during the first 12 years after spinal cord injury. Archives of physical medicine and rehabilitation. 1993;74:248.
26. DeVivo MJ. Causes and costs of spinal cord injury in the United States. Spinal cord. 1997;35(12):809-13.
27. Dijkers M. Quality of life after spinal cord injury: a meta analysis of the effects of disablement components. Spinal cord. 1997;35(12):829-40.
28. Ditunno JF, et al. The international standards booklet for neurological and functional classification of spinal cord injury. Spinal Cord. 1994;32(2):70-80.
29. Dykstra DD, et al. Effects of botulinum A toxin on detrusor-sphincter dyssynergia in spinal cord injury patients. The Journal of urology. 1988;139(5):919-22.
30. Elliott TR, Patricia R. Spinal Cord Injury. Handbook of psychology. 2003.
31. Emery E, et al. Apoptosis after traumatic human spinal cord injury. Journal of neurosurgery. 1998;89(6):911-20.
32. Essentials of Spinal Cord Injury: Basic Research to Clinical Practice By Michael.
33. Faden AI, Simon RP. A potential role for excitotoxins in the pathophysiology of spinal cord injury. Annals of neurology. 1988;23(6):623-6.
34. Faulkner JR, et al. Reactive astrocytes protect tissue and preserve function after spinal cord injury. The Journal of Neuroscience. 2004;24(9):2143-55.
35. Fehlings MG, Tator CH. The relationships among the severity of spinal cord injury, residual neurological function, axon counts, and counts of retrogradely labeled neurons after experimental spinal cord injury. Experimental neurology. 1995;132(2):220-8.
36. Frankel HL, et al. Long-term survival in spinal cord injury: a fifty year investigation. Spinal cord. 1998;36(4):266-74.
37. Fraser A, EDMONDS-SEAL J. Spinal Cord Injuries. Anesthesia. 1982;37(11):1084-98.
38. Gale K, Kerasidis H, Wrathall JR. Spinal cord contusion in the rat: behavioral analysis of functional neurologic impairment. Experimental neurology. 1985;88(1):123-34.

39. Grill R, et al. Cellular delivery of neurotrophin-3 promotes corticospinal axonal growth and partial functional recovery after spinal cord injury. The Journal of neuroscience. 1997;17(14): 5560-72.
40. Gruner JA. A monitored contusion model of spinal cord injury in the rat. Journal of neurotrauma. 1992;9(2):123-8.
41. Heinemann AW. Spinal Cord Injury. Handbook of health and rehabilitation psychology. Springer US. 1995;341-60.
42. How I Roll: Life, Love and work After a Spinal Cord Injury. By J Bryant Neville Jr.
43. Hurlbert RJ. Methylprednisolone for acute spinal cord injury: an inappropriate standard of care*. Journal of Neurosurgery: spine. 2000;93(1):1-7.
44. International standards for neurological and functional classification of spinal cord injury. American Spinal Injury Association. 1996.
45. Janssen TWJ, Maria TEH. Spinal cord injury. Exercise testing and exercise prescription for special cases: theoretical basis and clinical applications. 2005;203-19.
46. Kalsbeek WD, et al. The national head and spinal cord injury survey: major findings. Journal of Neurosurgery. 1980;S19-31.
47. Katz NM, et al. Incremental risk factors for spinal cord injury following operation for acute traumatic aortic transection. The Journal of thoracic and cardiovascular surgery. 1981;81(5): 669-74.
48. Keirstead HS, et al. Human embryonic stem cell-derived oligodendrocyte progenitor cell transplants remyelinate and restore locomotion after spinal cord injury. The Journal of Neuroscience. 2005;25(19):4694-4705.
49. Kraus JF, et al. Incidence of traumatic spinal cord lesions. Journal of chronic diseases. 1975;28(9):471-92.
50. Liu D, Wipawan T, McAdoo DJ. Excitatory amino acids rise to toxic levels upon impact injury to the rat spinal cord. Brain research. 1991;547(2):344-8.
51. Liu XZ, et al. Neuronal and glial apoptosis after traumatic spinal cord injury. The Journal of neuroscience. 1997;17(14):5395-406.
52. Lu P, et al. Neural stem cells constitutively secrete neurotrophic factors and promote extensive host axonal growth after spinal cord injury. Experimental neurology. 2003;181(2):115-29.

53. Marino RJ, et al. International standards for neurological classification of spinal cord injury. The journal of spinal cord medicine. 2003;26:S50.
54. Maynard FM, et al. International standards for neurological and functional classification of spinal cord injury. Spinal cord. 1997;35(5):266-74.
55. Mayo Clinic Guide to Living with a Spinal Cord Injury. By Mayo Clinic
56. McDonald JW, et al. Transplanted embryonic stem cells survive, differentiate and promote recovery in injured rat spinal cord. Nature medicine. 1999;5(12):1410-2.
57. McDonald WJ, Sadowsky C. "Spinal-cord injury." The Lancet. 2002;359(9304):417-25.
58. McKinley WO, et al. Long-term medical complications after traumatic spinal cord injury: a regional model systems analysis. Archives of physical medicine and rehabilitation. 1999;80(11):1402-10.
59. Meyer Jr, PR, et al. Spinal Cord Injury. Neurologic clinics. 1991;9(3):625-61.
60. Michael J, Krause JS, Daniel PL. Recent trends in mortality and causes of death among persons with spinal cord injury. Archives of physical medicine and rehabilitation. 1999;80(11):1411-9.
61. Naftchi NE, et al. Pituitary-testicular axis dysfunction in spinal cord injury. Spinal Cord Injury. Springer Netherlands. 1982; 243-52.
62. Neumann S, Woolf CJ. Regeneration of dorsal column fibers into and beyond the lesion site following adult spinal cord injury. Neuron. 1999;23(1):83-91.
63. Nobunaga AI, Bette KG, Rosalie BK. Recent demographic and injury trends in people served by the Model Spinal Cord Injury Care Systems. Archives of physical medicine and rehabilitation. 1999;80(11):1372-82.
64. Okada S, et al. Conditional ablation of Stat3 or Socs3 discloses a dual role for reactive astrocytes after spinal cord injury. Nature medicine. 2006;12(7):829-34.
65. Pang D, Wilberger JE. Spinal cord injury without radiographic abnormalities in children. Journal of neurosurgery. 1982;57(1):114-29.
66. Papadopoulos SM. Spinal Cord Injury. Current Opinion in Neurology. 1992;5(4):554-7.

67. Pearse DD, et al. cAMP and Schwann cells promote axonal growth and functional recovery after spinal cord injury. Nature medicine. 2004;10(6):610-6.
68. Pointillart V, et al. Pharmacological therapy of spinal cord injury during the acute phase. Spinal cord. 2000;38(2):71-6.
69. Popovich PG, et al. Depletion of hematogenous macrophages promotes partial hindlimb recovery and neuroanatomical repair after experimental spinal cord injury. Experimental neurology. 1999;158(2):351-65.
70. Popovich PG, Ping W, Bradford TS. Cellular inflammatory response after spinal cord injury in sprague-dawley and lewis rats. Journal of comparative neurology. 1997;377(3):443-64.
71. Proctor MR. Spinal Cord Injury. Critical care medicine. 2002;30(11):S489-S499.
72. Raineteau O, Schwab ME. Plasticity of motor systems after incomplete spinal cord injury. Nature Reviews Neuroscience. 2001;2(4):263-73.
73. Richards JS, Donald GK, Christopher AP. Spinal Cord Injury. Handbook of rehabilitation psychology. 2000;11-27.
74. Rivlin AS, Tator CH. Effect of duration of acute spinal cord compression in a new acute cord injury model in the rat. Surgical neurology. 1978;10(1):38-43.
75. Rivlin AS, Tator CH. Objective clinical assessment of motor function after experimental spinal cord injury in the rat. Journal of neurosurgery. 1977;47(4):577-81.
76. Ruge D. Spinal Cord Injuries. American Journal of Physical Medicine & Rehabilitation. 1971;50(1):42.
77. Sadowsky C, et al. "Spinal Cord Injury." Disability and Rehabilitation. 2002;24(13):680-7.
78. Schallert T, et al. CNS plasticity and assessment of forelimb sensorimotor outcome in unilateral rat models of stroke, cortical ablation, parkinsonism and spinal cord injury. Neuropharmacology. 2000;39(5):777-87.
79. Schneider RC, Glenn C, Pantek H. The syndrome of acute central cervical spinal cord injury; with special reference to the mechanisms involved in hyperextension injuries of cervical spine. Journal of neurosurgery. 1954;11(6):546-77.
80. Sekhon LHS, Michael GF. Epidemiology, demographics, and pathophysiology of acute spinal cord injury. Spine. 2001;26(24):S2-S12.

81. Short DJ, Masry WSE, Jones PW. High dose methylprednisolone in the management of acute spinal cord injury-a systematic review from a clinical perspective. Spinal cord. 2000;38(5): 273-86.
82. Siddall PJ, Taylor DA, Cousins MJ. Classification of pain following spinal cord injury. Spinal cord. 1997;35(2):69-75.
83. Spinal Cord Injuries: Management and Rehabilitation. By Sue Ann Sisto.
84. Spinal Cord Injury: A Guide to Living (A John Hopkins press book) Sara Palmer.
85. Spinal Cord Injury: Functional Rehabilitation. By Martha Freeman Somers.
86. Spinal Cord Injury and the Family: A New Guide (Howard University Press).
87. Spinal cord Medicine. By Denise I Campagnolo.
88. Springer JE, Azbill RD, Knapp PE. Activation of the caspase-3 apoptotic cascade in traumatic spinal cord injury. Nature medicine. 1999;5(8):943-6.
89. Standards for neurological and functional classification of spinal cord injury. American Spinal Injury Association. 1992.
90. Stover SL, DeLisa JA, Whiteneck GG, (eds). Spinal cord injury: clinical outcomes from the model systems. Aspen Publishers. 1995.
91. Stover SL, Kennedy EJ, Fine PR. Spinal cord injury: the facts and figures. University of Alabama at Birmingham. 1986.
92. Tator CH. Update on the pathophysiology and pathology of acute spinal cord injury. Brain Pathology. 1995;5(4):407-13.
93. Teng YD, et al. Functional recovery following traumatic spinal cord injury mediated by a unique polymer scaffold seeded with neural stem cells. Proceedings of the National Academy of Sciences. 2002;99(5):3024-9.
94. The Spinal Cord Injury Handbook: For Patients and Families. By Richard Senelick.
95. Westgren N, Levi R. Quality of life and traumatic spinal cord injury. Archives of physical medicine and rehabilitation. 1998;79(11):1433-9.
96. Whiteneck GG, et al. Mortality, morbidity, and psychosocial outcomes of persons spinal cord injured more than 20 years ago. Spinal Cord. 1992;30(9):617-30.

97. Wrathall JR, Pettegrew RK, Harvey F. Spinal cord contusion in the rat: production of graded, reproducible, injury groups. Experimental neurology. 1985;88(1):108-22.
98. Wyndaele M, Wyndaele JJ. Incidence, prevalence and epidemiology of spinal cord injury: what learns a worldwide literature survey?. Spinal cord. 2006;44(9):523-9.
99. Yekutiel M, et al. The prevalence of hypertension, ischaemic heart disease and diabetes in traumatic spinal cord injured patients and amputees. Spinal Cord. 1989;27(1):58-62.
100. Young W. Secondary injury mechanisms in acute spinal cord injury. The Journal of emergency medicine. 1992;11:13-22.

EXTERNAL LINKS

1. www.apparelyzed.com
2. www.brainandspinalcord.org
3. www.criminallawbaltimore.com
4. www.en.wikipedia.org/wiki/spinal-cord-injury
5. www.MageeRehab.org
6. www.mayoclinic.org/diseases-conditions/spinal-cord-injury/basics/....
7. www.medical-dictionary.thefreedictionary.com/spinal+cord+injury
8. www.medicinenet.comspinal_cord_injury_treatment_and.....
9. www.ninds.nih.gov/disorders/sci
10. www.spinalcord.org
11. www.spinal-cord.org/spinal-cord-injury.htm

Index

Page numbers followed by *f* refer to figure.

C

G

H

Q

R

S

W

X

Y

Z